Conjugal Love and Procreation

Conjugal Love and Procreation

Dietrich von Hildebrand's Superabundant Integration

Kevin Schemenauer

LEXINGTON BOOKS
Lanham • Boulder • New York • Toronto • Plymouth, UK

Published by Lexington Books
A wholly owned subsidiary of The Rowman & Littlefield Publishing Group, Inc.
4501 Forbes Boulevard, Suite 200, Lanham, Maryland 20706
http://www.lexingtonbooks.com

Estover Road, Plymouth PL6 7PY, United Kingdom

British Library Cataloguing in Publication Information Available

Library of Congress Cataloging-in-Publication Data
Schemenauer, Kevin, 1981–
Conjugal love and procreation : Dietrich von Hildebrand's superabundant integration / Kevin Schemenauer.
p. cm.
Includes bibliographical references (p.) and index.
ISBN 978-0-7391-4706-1 (cloth : alk. paper) — ISBN 978-0-7391-4708-5 (ebook)
1. Von Hildebrand, Dietrich, 1889–1977. 2. Sex—Religious aspects—Catholic Church. 3. Marriage—Religious aspects—Catholic Church. 4. Human reproduction—Religious aspects—Catholic Church. 5. Catholic Church—Doctrines. I. Title.
BX1795.S48S35 2011
241'.66—dc22 2011004684

™ The paper used in this publication meets the minimum requirements of American National Standard for Information Sciences—Permanence of Paper for Printed Library Materials, ANSI/NISO Z39.48-1992.

Printed in the United States of America

To my beloved, Frances Schemenauer

Children cannot live and grow humanly without . . . love.—Jean Vanier

Contents

Acknowledgments

The conception and rearing of this work was not the work of one individual but the fruit of many hands. The One who played the most important role is the Triune God who in Love created all things and established that procreation should overflow from the depths of conjugal love. My parents played a unique role by participating in the mystery of procreation and accepting the fruit of that mystery with loving care.

Although the manuscript has seen a number of revisions in the last few years, it was first a dissertation written at The Catholic University of America. Without the financial support of the university I would not have been able to pursue a Ph.D. in Moral Theology/Ethics, much less write this work. In particular, my dissertation director, John Grabowski, with his breadth of knowledge, eager use of red ink, and encouragement throughout my graduate studies has left a lasting impression on this manuscript and on my soul. Others who contributed in some way to the formulation of editing of this work include Andy Lichtenwalner, William Daniel, Damian Fedoryka, Michael Waldstein, Janet Smith, Brian Johnstone, Kenneth Schmitz, Sean Kinsella, and Mark Reasoner.

I owe a debt of gratitude to Dietrich von Hildebrand. This book is largely a synthesis and analysis of his rich insights. I had access and exposure to his thought in part because of the vigorous support that Alice von Hildebrand and The Dietrich von Hildebrand Legacy Project have given to Dietrich von Hildebrand's life, writing, and thought. Thanks to the Legacy Project, I had access to a comprehensive bibliography of von Hildebrand's works at the beginning of my research and was able to clarify my thinking at two von Hildebrand conferences. The Legacy project also granted me permission to quote extensively from four of von Hildebrand's works: *The Encyclical "Hu-*

manae Vitae": A Sign of Contradiction; *Man and Woman*; *Marriage*; and *Purity: The Mystery of Christian Spirituality*.

For help in the mature stages of this work, I am thankful to Holy Family Parish in Mitchellville, Maryland, Marian University, and Lexington Press. Holy Family Parish employed my wife, enabling me to work full-time on the dissertation for a year. Marian University employed me and supported my research with a Bonaventure Research Award. A special note of thanks goes to my department chair, Andy Hohman, for decreasing my course preparations for three semesters. I am thankful to Lexington Press for their willingness to support and publish this work. I appreciate the anonymous reviewer who suggested that I highlight more how von Hildebrand integrates conjugal love and procreation. Thank you also to Melissa Wilks and Jessica McCleary for leading the editing and publishing process.

Finally, I thank my wife, Frances, my son Gabriel, and the yet to be named superabundant fruit who likely will be born before this work goes to press. Although my wife has not read a single page of this manuscript, our shared conjugal love has motivated my interest in the topic and encouraged me to bring the project to a completion.

Introduction

In his work *Why God Became Man*, Saint Anselm writes that Adam was created from nothing, Eve from man alone, and all other humans from both man and woman. The one mode of creation that remained was the bringing forth of man out of woman alone, and this God reserved for the conception of His Son.[1] Anselm brings to light a distinguishing feature of creation, the Incarnation, and procreation. Dietrich von Hildebrand's account of marriage and the conjugal act highlights two key similarities of these three events. All three remind humanity of its place as a creature before the Creator and all three manifest God's superabundant love.

Compared to the extraordinary events of the world's creation and the Incarnation of the Son of God, procreation can seem ordinary—children are conceived everyday. One's familiarity with procreation may tempt one to deny the depth and mysterious character of this event and thereby approach the gift of new life in an unreflective manner. In the Judeo-Christian faith, however, procreation has had a central role in the ongoing covenantal relation between God and His people. Adam and Eve were instructed to: "Be fertile and multiply" (Gen. 1:28).[2] Abram, who would become the *father* of faith, and his wife Sarai, struggled with infertility even while God promised them descendants as numerous as the stars (Gen. 15:5).

Procreation remains central in the Church today. Differing understandings of marriage and the role of procreation in marriage are at the heart of many currently debated moral issues: overpopulation, under-population, natural family planning, contraception, in vitro fertilization, surrogacy, cloning, infertility, homosexual unions, abortion, frozen embryo adoption, and embryonic stem cell research. These debates concern, in one way or another, the manner in which marriage and the conjugal act relate to conjugal love and procreation. I do not intend to resolve these contemporary issues, but to clarify the relationship between conjugal love, procreation, and marriage through an analysis of Dietrich von Hildebrand's published writings.

Von Hildebrand's writings are important to discussion of marriage and the conjugal act for various reasons. The synthesis he brings to conjugal love and procreation in marriage approaches, perhaps closer than any other twentieth century thinker, the thought and writings of John Paul II. Von Hildebrand provides a profound, supportive, and distinct voice next to John Paul II's work, which has had to bear the weight in the last generation of integrating the centrality of conjugal love in marriage with Catholic sexual teaching.

Von Hildebrand's early writings influenced the Catholic tradition's growing recognition of conjugal love's role in marriage. This increased role of conjugal love, along with a host of other factors, led many in the mid-twentieth century to challenge Catholic sexual teaching. Catholic theologians and leaders struggled to articulate the integration of conjugal love and procreation in a way that was consistent with previous ecclesial statements. The events leading up to and following the publication of Paul VI's *Humanae vitae* are well documented.[3] Nonetheless, a brief survey of those events is necessary to highlight von Hildebrand's contemporary relevance.

Moral reflection had been dominated by a cold legalism for centuries and many Catholics grew to see Catholic sexual ethics as a list of what not to do, and an arbitrary list at that. Increased reflection on personal values and conjugal love led many to raise questions about contraception, abortion, and homosexual unions. Many Protestant bodies were changing their teaching on these issues.

Following the second Vatican council, the pope arranged a Pontifical Study Commission to study the issue of contraception. In light of other changes following Vatican II, many expected a change on contraception as well. The conclusion of the study commission was leaked to the public and the majority position was that the church's position should change. Many pastors went silent on the issue or began advising parishioners to follow their conscience. A few years later, Paul VI issued *Humanae vitae*. To the surprise of many, Paul VI maintained that contraceptive acts are always immoral and harmful for marriages. A number of national bishop conferences challenged or raised questions about *Humanae vitae*. In the United States, Charles Curran led a newspaper press conference the day after the encyclical's publication with a statement of dissent signed by eighty-seven theologians. Even many who agreed with the conclusion of *Humanae vitae* raised questions, as did the minority report of the Pontifical Study Commission, about the legitimacy of opposing contraceptive acts on the basis of traditional natural law arguments.

Karol Wojtyla, who would become John Paul II, was on the Pontifical Study Commission but was unable to attend the final meetings. He would spend a large portion of his papacy seeking to provide what was lacking in the study commission, an account of marriage that integrates conjugal love with the tradition's emphasis on procreation. The influence of John Paul II's writings on marriage in the last thirty years cannot be under-stated. John Paul II Institutes for Marriage and Family have opened in eight countries located on four continents. At least in the United States, popular and scholarly commentaries of John Paul II's writings on marriage and family, as well as presentations and discussion groups on the theology of the body, occur with a frequency second only to Bible commentaries and study groups.

A re-appropriation of von Hildebrand's writings would provide a parallel voice to the work of John Paul II. A dialogue between these two thinkers stands to bear great fruit. While von Hildebrand anticipates John Paul II in many ways, discussion of von Hildebrand's writings is not merely of historical interest. His writing has a vibrancy that speaks with an original voice to current concerns. In particular, von Hildebrand's rich analysis of conjugal love, procreation as a superabundant fruit of conjugal love, and the virtue of reverence each provide distinct and important considerations that would enrich contemporary discussion of Catholic sexual ethics.

In the late 1920s, von Hildebrand drew from his zeal for the Church and his phenomenological background to write his influential works, *Reinheit und Jungfräulichkeit* ("Purity and Virginity")[4] and *Die Ehe* ("Marriage").[5] He proposed that conjugal love is a unique form of love, a form of love that has central importance in marriage. Through these remarks, von Hildebrand contributed to the Church's growing appreciation of conjugal love's role in marriage.[6] Nonetheless, despite this contribution, the response to the German publication of these works was quiet approval.[7] Similarly, von Hildebrand's "Lambeth-Botschaft," a response article to the 1930 Lambeth Conference, also received little to no commentary.[8]

One thinker who noticed von Hildebrand's work on marriage was Herbert Doms. Six years after von Hildebrand's *Die Ehe*, Doms wrote *Vom Sinn und Zweck der Ehe* ("On the Meaning and End of Marriage").[9] Doms mentions von Hildebrand's work in his introduction and then states that von Hildebrand did not go far enough in arguing for the centrality of love in marriage. Doms writes, "This emphasis on marriage as a community rather than as merely an institution to reproduce and educate children has for centuries been part of the teaching of many thinkers inside the Catholic Church."[10] Unlike the quiet reaction to von Hildebrand's work, Doms's book ignited large scale debate.[11]

Unfortunately, von Hildebrand did not participate in these debates. He had raised vocal opposition to the Nazi party and fled Munich for his life when the Nazis gained control of Germany in 1933.[12] Then, from 1933-1938, he edited an anti-Nazi weekly, *Der Christliche Ständesstaat* in Vienna.[13] After the Anschluß, he fled again. Two years later, he left Europe altogether and finally set down roots in New York.

Von Hildebrand did not publish on marriage and sexual ethics again until 1942 when he collaborated with two other scholars to translate his work *Die Ehe* into English. The English version received significantly more commentary than did the original. The different response to his work is an indication of the wider readership that von Hildebrand's writings would receive in the United States.[14] Perhaps, more importantly, however, the 1942 English translation of *Die Ehe* was published amid growing controversy surrounding both the German (1935) and English (1939) publication of Doms's *Vom Sinn und Zweck der Ehe*.[15] Since the English translation of *Die Ehe* is published three years after the English translation of Doms's work, controversy surrounding the latter's work influenced discussion of the former.[16]

The continuity of von Hildebrand's thought on marriage is impressive in light of the fact that after his "Lambeth-Botschaft" article, he did not publish another work on the subject for thirty-five years. His next related publication is his 1966, *Man and Woman*, a collection of essays treating marriage and the distinction between the sexes.[17] Two years later, he published a defense of *Humanae vitae* entitled, *Die Enzyklika "Humanae Vitae": Ein Zeichen des Wiederspruchs*, which was translated into English in 1969 as *The Encyclical "Humanae Vitae": A Sign of Contradiction*.[18] Then, he published *Zölibat und Glaubenskrise* in 1970, translated into English as *Celibacy and the Crisis of Faith* in 1971.[19] Finally, in 1971, von Hildebrand published the culmination of his reflection on love, *Das Wesen der Liebe* ("The Nature of Love"). This latter work was translated into English in 2009.[20]

The most significant commentary on von Hildebrand's thought on marriage dates from no earlier than the mid-1980s. The emphasis of the commentary has been to highlight von Hildebrand's contribution to the Catholic tradition's growing recognition of the role of spousal love, and thereby the unitive aspect of marriage. In 1986, Geoffrey Grubb wrote a dissertation titled "The Anthropology of Marriage in Significant Roman Catholic Documents from *Casti Connubii* to *Gaudium et Spes* (Doms, Hildebrand)."[21] This work discusses the context and content of Pius XI's *Casti connubii* and then highlights the writings of both Dietrich von Hildebrand and Herbert Doms. The work concludes with commentary on the marriage section of *Gaudium et spes*. Grubb's work provides a brief but excellent summary of von Hildebrand's thought on conjugal love and marriage and summarizes well the immediate reaction to his early works.

In 1996, Rolando Arjonillo completed a dissertation titled, "Conjugal Love and the Ends of Marriage in Dietrich von Hildebrand and Herbert Doms: A Review and Appraisal in the Light of *Gaudium et Spes*."[22] The outline of Arjonillo's work is remarkably similar to that of Grubb's earlier work. Arjonillo, however, spends relatively little time on *Casti connubii* and provides more consideration of the philosophical background and anthropological foundations for the thought of von Hildebrand and Doms. Further,

Arjonillo's dissertation was published in book form in 1998 and accordingly has received greater exposure.[23]

Grubb and Arjonillo provide nice summaries of von Hildebrand's account of conjugal love in relation to *Gaudium et spes*. I intend to engage and build on their research by also focusing on von Hildebrand's published thought on procreation's role in marriage. In particular, I intend to examine more closely the relationship between von Hildebrand's treatment of conjugal love and his treatment of procreation. Both Grubb and Arjonillo argue that despite von Hildebrand's emphasis on conjugal love, von Hildebrand did not invert the traditional hierarchy of ends in marriage. I aim to take this conclusion a step further. I propose that von Hildebrand's treatment of conjugal love clarifies and enhances procreation's role in marriage.

I argue this thesis on the basis of two themes central to von Hildebrand's thought: reverence and superabundance. One can understand, his analysis of procreation only in light of these two important concepts. My only qualification of this thesis is that von Hildebrand does not offer a developed notion of the God-entrusted spousal mission to have and raise children. Even here, his general framework, and especially his affirmation that conception should be postponed only for serious reasons, implies that spouses have a mission to raise and educate children. I highlight how his account complements the Catholic tradition's emphasis on the good of children through comparisons with Augustine and Aquinas and more recent statements made by Pius XII, the Fathers of Vatican Two, Paul VI, and John Paul II.

While my central concern is to investigate the relationship between conjugal love and procreation in marriage through the lens of von Hildebrand, a further intention is to describe systematically von Hildebrand's account of marriage and sexual ethics. Von Hildebrand's style of presentation is both a blessing and an obstacle for those who study his writings. On the topic of marriage, his poetic language and manner of unfolding the distinguishing features of marriage testifies to the mysterious nature of marriage. Yet, with his poetic presentation comes an occasional lack of clarity in his use of key terms and distinctions. I seek to analyze the consistency of his writings and the validity of his key terms and distinctions, knowingly risking, but certainly not intending, the loss of beauty and appreciation of marriage's mystery as found in his writings.

Although I seek to provide a systematic account of von Hildebrand's published writings, my aim is not merely to write what another has written. I focus on von Hildebrand's writings because they shed light on the reality of things. In treating his writings systematically, I work through tensions that he does not directly address. In this, I make small additions to von Hildebrand's writings.

I approach von Hildebrand's remarks on conjugal love and procreation in marriage in two parts. Each part has three chapters. The first part deals with conjugal love, marriage, and the conjugal act. In the first chapter, I summarize his reflections on conjugal love, natural marriage, and the uniqueness of conjugal love and marriage in a Christian framework. While Grubb and Arjonillo have already provided similar analyses, I begin with a summary of von Hildebrand's remarks on marriage because I presume this foundation in my account of procreation. Further, in distinction to these previous works, my summary is more thorough than that of Grubb's, more in line with von Hildebrand's order of presentation than that of Arjonillo's, and includes a broader engagement with both the later works of von Hildebrand as well as the available commentary on von Hildebrand's work. This chapter relies heavily on von Hildebrand's *Marriage*.

In my summary, I intentionally systematize von Hildebrand's remarks in two ways. First, I follow the twofold division of his work, *Marriage*, into natural conjugal love and marriage and the transformation of conjugal love and marriage in the light of Christ. By natural marriage, I understand that von Hildebrand means what could be known of marriage without God's intervening grace and revelation. Accordingly, although he quotes Scripture and liturgical prayers in his account of natural marriage, I reserve these quotations for my summary of his presentation on sacramental marriage. Similarly, when he develops aspects of conjugal love and marriage in a manner that does not rely on Christian revelation, I add the remarks to his discussion of conjugal love and natural marriage. Despite these occasional exceptions and some supplementary material that I add from his other works, I generally follow the order of presentation found in his work *Marriage*.

In the second chapter, I summarize von Hildebrand's remarks on the conjugal act. He argues that the action is essentially deep because it is an actualization of conjugal love and the consummation of marriage. As distinguished from his treatment of marriage, von Hildebrand does not dedicate a work solely to the topic of the conjugal act. Accordingly, although I draw heavily from his earlier work, *Purity*, I do not follow the structure of any one of his works, but pull significantly from various works.

In chapter three, I discuss von Hildebrand's proposal that conjugal love is the primary meaning of marriage. I engage and summarize commentary of this proposal and I explain different ways that one could apply the phrase "primary meaning" to von Hildebrand's remarks on conjugal love. I contend that von Hildebrand does not explicitly define what he means by this phrase. However, I propose with Rolando Arjonillo that he implicitly means that conjugal love is the authentic motivation for and vitality of marriage. Chapter three draws heavily on *Marriage*.

The second part is more focused on procreation and attempts to show how von Hildebrand integrates conjugal love and procreation in marriage. In chapter four, I analyze the principle of superabundance and the virtue of reverence. In light of these concepts, I argue that procreation is the primary end of marriage because it deals with one's fundamental disposition before God. From here, I contend that von Hildebrand's account of conjugal love enhances procreation's role in marriage in two ways. First, conjugal love (and the lover's reverence for the beloved, marriage, and the conjugal act implied therein) encourages reverence for procreation. Second, his emphasis on conjugal love highlights the idea that procreation, like creation, is rooted in love. This chapter draws on a number of von Hildebrand's works. In particular, the discussion of reverence draws from *Liturgy and Personality* and his account of superabundant finality from *The Encyclical "Humanae Vitae"* and *The Nature of Love*.

In the fifth and sixth chapters, I examine how von Hildebrand applies his general remarks on spousal love and procreation to the rhythm method and artificial birth control. While not engaging the whole theological discussion of these issues, this analysis is conducted in light of Pius XII's address, "The Apostolate of the Midwife," *Gaudium et spes*, *Humanae vitae*, all written late in von Hildebrand's career and *Familiaris consortio*, written five years after von Hildebrand's death.

In the fifth chapter, I connect von Hildebrand's account of the rhythm method with his previous analysis of conjugal love. While von Hildebrand's writings lack a developed notion of the parental mission to conceive and educate children, his analysis of conjugal love and procreation does more than simply avoid contradicting Catholic moral teaching. His writings provide a well cultivated ground from which Catholic sexual ethics can flourish. In chapter five, I outline his distinction between two different understandings of the term "nature" and his response to those who argue that the abstinence required by the rhythm method is too great of a burden for spouses to endure. Von Hildebrand's *Die Enzyklika "Humanae Vitae"* and *Man and Woman*, as well as his article, "Lambeth-Botschaft," are vital in chapter five as they are in chapter six.

The last chapter deals with von Hildebrand's analysis of artificial birth control. Von Hildebrand responds to the claim that artificial birth control is necessary to promote conjugal love. He argues that use of artificial birth control is a grave sin of irreverence and thereby undermines authentic conjugal love. The chapter ends with von Hildebrand's discussion of conscience and the role that conscience should play in spousal discernment of the appropriate means for postponing pregnancy. Finally, the conclusion offers a general summary with emphasis on unique contributions that von Hildebrand offers and topics for further study.

Notes

1. Saint Anselm, *Why God Became Man and the Virgin Conception and Original Sin*, trans. Joseph Colleran (Albany, NY: Magi Books, 1969), 126-28.
2. All Scripture quotations are taken from the New American Bible.

3. For more details on this history, see John Grabowski, *Sex and Virtue: An Introduction to Sexual Ethics* (Washington, D.C.: The Catholic University of America, 2003), 1-22; William H. Shannon, *The Lively Debate: Response to Humanae Vitae* (New York: Sheed and Ward, 1970); John T. Noonan, *Contraception: A History of Its Treatment by the Catholic Theologians and Canonists*, 2nd ed. (Cambridge, MA: Harvard University Press, 1986).

4. Dietrich von Hildebrand, *Reinheit und Jungfräulichkeit* (Cologne: Oratoriums Verlag, 1927). This work was first translated into English as *In Defense of Purity: An Analysis of the Catholic Ideals of Purity and Virginity* (New York: Longmans, Green and Co., 1931). The translator is not listed. I am using a reprint of the original English translation, *Purity: The Mystery of Christian Sexuality* (Steubenville, OH: Franciscan University Press, 1989). This reprint also fails to list the name of the translator.

5. Dietrich von Hildebrand, *Die Ehe* (Munich: Verlag Ars Sacra, 1929), trans. Dietrich von Hildebrand, Emmanuel Chapman, and Daniel Sullivan as *Marriage* (London: Longmans, Green, 1942). Von Hildebrand's work, *Die Ehe*, is first said to have been published in 1929 by every source except a bibliography provided by a well-known student of von Hildebrand, Balduin Schwarz, who states that the work was first published in 1928 (Balduin Schwarz, ed., *The Human Person and the World of Values: A Tribute to Dietrich von Hildebrand by His Friends in Philosophy* [New York: Fordham University Press, 1960], 196). Note that two sentences from *Die Ehe*, 37-38, are not directly translated into English. These sentences, which deal with the relationship between conjugal love and marriage's indissolubility, are re-formulated in the English edition and mixed with an added discussion of the risks and sacrifices of marriage (*Marriage*, 49-52).

6. John Noonan, in his historical analysis of contraception as treated in the Catholic tradition, writes that von Hildebrand was "the first married layman to make a substantial contribution to Catholic doctrine on marriage. . . . For the first time, a Catholic writer taught that love was a requirement of lawful, marital coition" (John T. Noonan, Jr., *Contraception: A History of Its Treatment by the Catholic Theologians and Canonists*, 2nd ed. [Cambridge, MA: Harvard University Press, 1986], 494-95); see also William H. Shannon, *The Lively Debate: Response to 'Humanae Vitae'* (New York: Sheed and Ward, 1970), 17-22; Theodore Mackin, S.J., *What Is Marriage?* (New York: Paulist Press, 1982), 225-29; John S. Grabowski, *Sex and Virtue: An Introduction to Sexual Ethics* (Washington, DC: The Catholic University of America Press, 2003), 11, 85-88; Alice von Hildebrand, *The Soul of a Lion* (San Francisco, CA: Ignatius Press, 2000), 212. Dietrich von Hildebrand notes the acknowledgment of his contribution in his preface to the English translation of *Marriage*: "It is perhaps permissible to say that [the present work's] influence, especially in its Italian and French translations, has been credited with bringing about an increased stress on the role of love in Christian marriage" (vi-vii).

7. Geoffrey Grubb, "The Anthropology of Marriage in Significant Roman Catholic Documents from *Casti Connubii* to *Gaudium et Spes* (Doms, Hildebrand)," PhD diss., Saint Louis University, 1986, 128-34.

8. Dietrich von Hildebrand, "Lambeth-Botschaft,"*Religiöse Besinnung* 4, 1 (1931/32): 20-29. This article is also included in a collection of von Hildebrand's articles: *Die Menschheit am Scheideweg: Gesammelte Abhandlungen und Vorträge*, ed. Karla Mertens (Regensburg: Josef Habbel, 1955), 146-57.

9. Herbert Doms, *Vom Sinn und Zweck der Ehe* (Breslau: Ostdeutsche Verlagsanstalt, 1935), trans. George Sayer as *The Meaning of Marriage* (London: Sheed and Ward, 1939).

10. *The Meaning of Marriage*, xvi.

11. Geoffrey Grubb describes the debates following Doms's work as resulting from Doms's "lack of tact in dealing with Thomism, his fundamental question concerning the nature of human sexual intercourse and the popularity of his book" (Grubb, 184; see also 182-83).

12. *The Soul of a Lion*, 236.

13. For a (slightly incomplete) collection of the articles von Hildebrand wrote for this weekly as well as his memoirs during this time see *Memoiren und Aufsätze gegen den Nationalsozialismus*, ed. Ernst Wenisch, Rudolf Ebneth, and Alice von Hildebrand (Mainz: Matthias-Grünewald, 1994).

14. Von Hildebrand's *Liturgy and Personality* received at least twenty book reviews in the two years following its English translation. Dietrich von Hildebrand, *Liturgy and Personality*,

trans. anonymous (New York: Longmans, Green, 1943). This work was originally published in German as *Liturgie und Persönlichkeit* (Salzburg: Anton Pustet, 1933). The edition I am using is *Liturgy and Personality*, rev. ed. (Baltimore: Helicon Press, 1960). Again, the translator is not listed.

15. For discussion of this debate, see Grubb, 134-84. Some of the tensest moments of the debates surround a decree of the Holy Office on April 1, 1944 which states that denying the primacy of procreation in marriage or the subordinate character of the secondary ends is inadmissible (*AAS* 36 [1944]: 103).

16. Bernard Lonergan writes in a review of von Hildebrand's *Marriage*, "the movement originating with von Hildebrand not only has not been condemned but, in the opinion of perhaps all writers in theological reviews, contains elements that are destined to enrich Catholic thought. On the other hand, the most downright [sic] member of this school, Dr. Herbert Doms, whose *Von Sinn und Zweck der Ehe* was published incompletely in English as *The Meaning of Marriage* (Sheed and Ward), received a very deliberate though unofficial rebuke from the Master of the Holy Office; and while von Hildebrand carefully avoids not only the more venturesome formulae but even the very name of Doms, it remains that he shares in the latter's fundamental outlook" (Bernard Lonergan, review of *Marriage*, by Dietrich von Hildebrand, in *Shorter Papers*, vol. 20 of *Collected Works of Bernard Lonergan*, ed. Frederick Crowe and Robert Doran [Toronto: University of Toronto Press, 2007], 155. One reviewer even mistakenly thinks that von Hildebrand wrote *Die Ehe* after Doms's work (M.P.B., review of *Marriage*, by Dietrich von Hildebrand, *Dominicana* 27 [October 1942]: 189).

17. Dietrich von Hildebrand, *Man and Woman* (Chicago: Franciscan Herald Press, 1966).

18. Dietrich von Hildebrand, *Die Enzyklika "Humanae Vitae": Ein Zeichen des Widerspruchs* (Regensburg: Josef Habbel, 1968), trans. Damian Fedoryka and John Crosby as *The Encyclical "Humanae Vitae": A Sign of Contradiction* (Chicago: Franciscan Herald Press, 1969).

19. Dietrich von Hildebrand, *Zölibat und Glaubenskrise* (Regensburg: Josef Habbel, 1970), trans. John F. Crosby as *Celibacy and the Crisis of Faith* (Chicago: Franciscan Herald Press, 1971).

20. Dietrich von Hildebrand, *Das Wesen der Liebe*, vol. 3 of *Dietrich von Hildebrand Gesammelte Werke*, ed. Dietrich von Hildebrand Gesellschaft (Regensburg: Josef Habbel, 1971), trans. John F. Crosby as *The Nature of Love* (South Bend, IN: St. Augustine's Press, 2009). John Crosby's translation of this work was done in collaboration with the Dietrich von Hildebrand Legacy Project which seeks to translate the remaining works of von Hildebrand not yet available in English. One can find more information about the Legacy Project at http://www.hildebrandlegacy.org.

21. Geoffrey Grubb, "The Anthropology of Marriage in Significant Roman Catholic Documents from *Casti Connubii* to *Gaudium et Spes* (Doms, Hildebrand)," PhD diss., Saint Louis University, 1986.

22. Rolando Arjonillo, "Conjugal Love and the Ends of Marriage in Dietrich von Hildebrand and Herbert Doms: a review and appraisal at the light of *Gaudium et Spes*," PhD diss., University of Navarre, 1997.

23. Rolando B. Arjonillo, *Conjugal Love of the Ends of Marriage: A Study of Dietrich von Hildebrand and Herbert Doms in the Light of the Pastoral Constitution 'Gaudium et Spes'* (Bern: Lang, 1998). I also should note two completed works that I was unable to access. The first work is a thesis written by Maria Dimpfl, titled "Das Wesen der ehelichen Liebe in Werken Dietrich von Hildebrands." Mag., Lateran Pontifical University in Rome, 1992-93. The second work is Joanna Sośnicka's dissertation entitled, "What Is the Essence of Love? Philosophical Analysis Based on the Thought of Dietrich von Hildebrand," PhD diss., International Academy of Philosophy in Liechtenstein, 2005.

Part I

Conjugal Love and Marriage

Chapter One

Conjugal Love and Marriage

Von Hildebrand divides his small treatise, *Marriage*, into two parts. In the first half, he distinguishes conjugal love from other forms of love and discusses the character of natural marriage. In the second half, he analyzes the Christian transformation of conjugal love and sacramental marriage.[1] My summary of his remarks on conjugal love and marriage follow this same order of presentation.

A. CONJUGAL LOVE

Von Hildebrand consistently begins his treatment of marriage with an analysis of conjugal love.[2] In his early work, *Marriage*, he devoted the first quarter of the book to conjugal love. He highlights this emphasis even more, forty years later, when von Hildebrand writes in his work, *The Encyclical "Humanae Vitae"*: "The very meaning and value which marriage possesses, of its own cannot be understood if we fail to start from the central reality of the love between man and woman."[3] In order to summarize von Hildebrand's account of marriage, therefore, one must begin with the distinctive character of conjugal love.

At the foundation of von Hildebrand's remarks on conjugal love is his affirmation that the one who has conjugal love is concerned not merely with particular features of the beloved, such as her social status or physical appearance, but with her complete personality.[4] On this point, one better understands von Hildebrand's analysis within the framework of his broader moral philosophy, that is, a realist ethics of value response. His basic assumption is that God created the world and established a created order. One must be attentive to created being as it reveals itself in everyday life. One must seek to understand both the content of individual things and the place of these things in the created order. Although one, at times, may fail to grasp certain things, this simply means that one must both recognize his limitations and strive ever more fully to understand the world around him. The moral agent must foster contact with the values of reality and then respond accordingly. A thing's values are those characteristics that remain good regardless of whether a human person appreciates them or not; the object's goodness is not merely good for someone, but good in itself. In the case of conjugal love, the foundational value is the beloved's complete personality.[5]

The beloved's personality becomes thematic, that is, the conscious focus of the lover. Von Hildebrand writes, "The beloved person is the object of our thoughts, sentiments, will, hope and longing; the beloved becomes the centre of our life, as far as created goods are concerned."[6] The lover gives a priority, in focus of attention and in energy exerted, to the beloved's well-being that he does not give to others. The lover's commitment to the beloved requires sacrifices of other urgent or deeply valuable goods.[7]

Von Hildebrand proposes that, in some cases, the lover grasps the beloved's personality at first sight. Conjugal love "can arise quite suddenly, and even develop to maturity at the first encounter of two persons."[8] Here, von Hildebrand avoids the error that conjugal love is a shallow infatuation by rooting it in the lovers' complete personalities.[9] He compares natural conjugal love to supernatural love of neighbor:

> Just as in supernatural love of our neighbor we penetrate at one glance to that innermost, mysterious essence of the other person in which, through all his imperfections, pettiness, arrogance, and triviality, he reflects God—in natural conjugal love the real individuality of the partner is mysteriously revealed; the deep, secret meaning which permeates all his gifts and talents, the whole rhythm of his being, is disclosed at one glance through all his imperfections. One understands, so to speak, the divine plan underlying the creation of this particular *individuality.*[10]

Even in natural conjugal love, the lover sees a glimpse of God's plan for the beloved. In this way, the lover has a bold vision of who the beloved ought to be. This vision looks past the beloved's sins, although not in the sense of failing to recognize the beloved's faults.[11] Rather, as von Hildebrand writes, "love is that which *gives us sight*, revealing to us even the faults of the other in their full import and causing us to suffer because of them."[12]

A second characteristic of conjugal love is mutuality. In fact, von Hildebrand argues that conjugal love is uniquely mutual: "there is an aspiration not merely for a return of affection in general, but for the unique love whereby the beloved belongs to the lover in an entirely exclusive manner, as he in turn wants to belong to the beloved."[13] This desire for mutual belonging orients conjugal love toward a unique union.[14]

Von Hildebrand proposes that every type of love has two features: "the desire for union with the beloved, the *intentio unionis*, and in the interest in the happiness or welfare of the loved one, the *intentio benevolentia*."[15] He argues that in each love, either the *intentio unionis* or the *intentio benevolentia* is more predominant. For conjugal love, the *intentio unionis* is primary. In fact, among natural forms of love, conjugal love involves the most profound unity: "the *intentio unionis* which is common to all categories of love assumes here not only its highest 'tension,' but also extends much farther than in any other love. We long for union with his very being; we long for a common life with him."[16]

Von Hildebrand explains this desire for union by distinguishing between *we* relationships and *I-thou* relationships. He writes: "In an I-thou communion, we are, as it were, in front of the other person and we look at each other. In the 'we communion,' on the contrary, we look together with the other person at some object."[17] Von Hildebrand maintains that among earthly relationships, conjugal love is the deepest form of an *I-thou* relation.[18] This emphasis on the unity of conjugal love is a theme that von Hildebrand retains throughout his career. Even into the 1960s, when theologians gave more consideration to the importance of love in marriage, von Hildebrand decried the fact that many Catholic authors failed to remark on the desire for union characteristic of conjugal love.[19]

For von Hildebrand, the intimate union of conjugal love can exist only between a man and a woman.[20] He maintains that men and women "represent two different types of mankind" and that this "metaphysical difference" gives men and women a unique capacity to complement one another.[21] He is careful to show, however, that the *general* complementarity of men and women does not prevent the fact that conjugal love is love of a *particular person*. The lover, then, sees the beloved not merely as a good representative of the other sex, but as individually embodying the charm of that sex.[22]

Accordingly, conjugal love is not simply friendship with someone of the complementary sex plus sensuality. He exclaims that sensual expression among friends who do not share conjugal love is morally repugnant.[23] He writes, "Only in conjugal love, where man and woman are united in a unique communion, where they give themselves to one another in the deepest sense of the word, and belong to each other in an ultimate interpenetration of their souls, does this relation to the sensual sphere become intelligible."[24] Sensual desire does not provide the framework from which to understand conjugal love, rather conjugal love provides the context necessary for understanding sensual desire.

In conjugal love, the lovers' deep respect for the other's personality, the making of the other thematic, and the mutual desire for intimate union, is correspondingly characterized by a distinct decisiveness. Von Hildebrand proposes that the decision to love another conjugally, unlike the possible uncertainty of whether someone is one's friend, can be answered with a clear "yes" or "no." This is not to say that one should jump into conjugal love unreflectively.[25] On the contrary, the decisiveness of one's love is an indication of that love's authenticity. If one remains uncertain about one's love, then one does not yet possess conjugal love. For von Hildebrand, this definite decision is expressed in the words "I love you." He states that "to add anything to those words and to say, 'I love you very much' . . . would be to lessen the force of the declaration."[26]

Further evidence of this decisive character is the intention for duration that conjugal love implies. While von Hildebrand acknowledges that one may think one shares conjugal love with another and then later realize this was not true, he affirms that the experience of this love necessarily entails an intention for the love's duration.[27] He writes, "Anyone who says, 'I am in love with this person now but I do not know whether I shall like him later on,' is not really in love."[28]

The lovers, motivated by their desire for mutual belonging and confident in the permanent character of their conjugal love, are able to give themselves to one another in a unique manner. Von Hildebrand writes, "the giving is literally complete and ultimate. Not only the heart but the entire personality is given up to the other."[29] This unique and mutual gift of self leads to a belonging among the lovers that excludes other parties.[30] Von Hildebrand writes: "The characteristics of complete mutual self-giving, and of being exclusively turned toward the beloved . . . exclude in themselves the possibility that this love can be directed simultaneously to more than one person."[31]

One should not confuse the beloved's belonging to the lover with egotistic possessiveness. Von Hildebrand illustrates the difference by comparing the possessiveness of a harem-owner with the self-giving characteristic of conjugal love.[32] Rather than leading to egotism, conjugal love has a positive and transforming influence on the lovers: "Being in love always implies a respectful, chivalrous attitude toward the beloved—a certain element of humility even, a melting of the soul, of the rigidity of the Ego. A person truly in love becomes tender and even *pure*."[33] Rather than leading the lover to close in on himself, conjugal love opens the lover to the world.

Von Hildebrand's rich analysis of conjugal love sheds light on the beauty of marriage and the appropriate motivations for entering marriage. While he maintains that "conjugal love is not yet marriage," he proposes that those who have authentic conjugal love will desire the consent of marriage and the permanent bond implied therein.[34] He writes, "marriage is precisely the fulfillment of this love."[35]

B. NATURAL MARRIAGE

Von Hildebrand's remarks on natural marriage highlight two themes: the relationship between conjugal love and marriage and the solemn character of marriage. He clarifies the relationship between conjugal love and marriage in his discussion of the true motivations for marriage. He repeatedly affirms that conjugal love is the fully adequate motivation for marriage. However, in addition to his discussion of the *fully adequate* motivation for marriage, he also remarks on other *morally legitimate* motivations:

> Although [conjugal] love is the real and adequate motive for concluding a marriage, this does not mean that all other motives are morally unworthy. . . . By this we mean a love which is not based on this unique, gladdening interpenetration of souls, this conviction of being destined for each other, but which is penetrated by a deep esteem for the partner and animated by the intention of forming a noble community of life. . . . Many people also are too coarse, too blunt, too primitive to experience such an ultimate conjugal love. They may, nevertheless, conclude marriage—although they only experience a more superficial love.[36]

Von Hildebrand presents a compelling vision of conjugal love as a model and inspiration, but does not commit himself to a false idealism that would require an actualization of this vision in every marital relationship.

If spouses need not embody conjugal love to enter marriage in a morally legitimate manner, then what is required? Von Hildebrand proposes that one characteristic of conjugal love must be present. He writes, "All motives not concerned with the other person as such . . . are completely unworthy."[37] The couple must at least have the seeds of conjugal love, namely, respect for the beloved. When this mutual respect is not present, then the contracting of marriage is immoral. For example, sensual desire absent of conjugal love is an inadmissible motivation. Such a motivation is selfish, degrading, impersonal, and undermines the solemn bond of marriage.[38]

Von Hildebrand also challenges the notion of "reasonable marriages." He writes,

> The so-called marriage of reason, which is decided after a cold calculation that one's financial situation can be improved and certain professional advantages attained, that both are peaceful and will get on together, that the ages are well suited—the marriage where such considerations instead of conjugal love constitute the motivation, where there is no longing for an indissoluble community with the beloved, is not only deprived of all beauty and plenitude, but is also something definitely *unreasonable*.[39]

The personality of the other, not sensual desire or professional advancement, serves as the worthy foundation for marriage.

Von Hildebrand proposes that in entering marriage, spouses commit themselves to fostering conjugal love toward one another. He writes, "love is called for from both spouses once marriage is completed . . . the fact that the other is the groom or bride presents a motive for love."[40] And yet, even though marriage is a motivation for developing conjugal love, the foundational motive for conjugal love remains the person of the beloved.[41]

While conjugal love anticipates marriage, the mere presence of conjugal love does not confer the sacrament. Marriage is "constituted only by a solemn act and presupposes a formal act of the will: the two partners give themselves expressly to each other, fully sanctioning this surrender for their entire lifetime."[42] Marital consent is a type of action which generates an objective bond not easily resolved.[43] The formal act of the will found in marital consent is like a promise or the enactment of legislation by a legitimate authority. In each case, formal actions create "an *objective reality* independent of the person."[44] However, whereas an act of legislation can be revised or even reversed, the formal commitment of marriage establishes an "objective bond, which once established, is withdrawn from the sphere of arbitrary decision of the persons concerned."[45]

Marital consent gives the spousal relationship a new status. The spouses, in entering marriage, prevent the contracting of marriage with others but also mutually promise to foster a more profound relationship of love with each other. Von Hildebrand writes,

> To maintain conjugal love in its entire grandeur and purity, in its glow, its depth and its vital plenitude is a task that arises for both partners with the conclusion of their marriage. It is difficult always to keep before us in all its same clarity and splendour the image of the other person so wonderfully revealed by love; because our laziness, our dullness, our constant falling back into periphery stultifies our vision. We should and must fight against this, for it constitutes a sin against the temple which we erected in our marriage.[46]

The new status of marriage demands that spouses promote conjugal love even when sacrifices and renewed commitments are required. This responsibility remains even if the partners' attitudes change for the worse.[47]

Von Hildebrand also remarks on the link between natural marriage and procreation. He writes, "Certainly, there is no greater mystery in the natural order of things than the fact that this closest of all unions procreates a human being with an immortal soul."[48] I am reserving further discussion of the relationship between marriage and procreation for a later chapter. Now, I turn to the Christian transformation of conjugal love and marriage.

C. THE TRANSFORMATION OF CONJUGAL LOVE

While von Hildebrand maintains that commitment to Christ does not eliminate but transfigures created nature, he also affirms that failure to consider creation from a Christian framework involves a "betrayal, a refusal to testify to the new light."[49] Conjugal love, when viewed in the light of Christ, retains its natural characteristics: concern for the complete personality of the beloved, thematic focus on the beloved, mutual, intending unity, between a man and a woman, decisive, intending duration, self-giving, and exclusive.[50] Nevertheless, conjugal love "assumes a completely new depth . . . in those persons who see everything consciously in the sight of God, who are aware that all things acquire an authentic importance only in Jesus and through Jesus, and who consider their own sanctification and that of others for the glory of God as the primordial, true task of man."[51] Von Hildebrand highlights three ways in which the lovers' disposition toward the beloved is transformed in Christ: the perception of the beloved's value, concern for the beloved, and the decreased temptation of making the beloved an idol.

In natural conjugal love, the lover aims to view the beloved not merely in terms of particular characteristics but in his complete personality. This holistic view is more fully accomplished in the light of Christ. Only in God does the lover view the beloved as a "being created by God," as made in the "image of God," and only in Christ is the beloved viewed as containing "an immortal soul redeemed by the blood of Jesus," as "loved by Jesus with an infinite and eternal love," as being "a temple of the Holy Ghost," as "destined to eternal communion with God," as "a vessel of grace," and as a "member of the Mystical Body of Christ."[52] Since the beloved's value is foundational in conjugal love, the dignity of man as revealed in Christ transforms this love at its roots.

Dedication to Christ also deepens the lover's concern for the beloved's well-being. The lover seeks not only the earthly good of the beloved but the beloved's eternal welfare. The salvation of the beloved, above all others, becomes the conscious concern of the lover.[53] The lover's concern for the beloved's eternal welfare becomes central in conjugal love and gives this love "a touching selflessness which is not possessed even by the highest natural love."[54]

While Christ illuminates the beloved's dignity and true well-being, He also makes clear the beloved's limitations. The lover's focus on the beloved in natural conjugal love risks making the beloved into an idol, a risk banished in supernatural conjugal love.[55] Since the love is centered on the one, true, God, the beloved is recognized as a being called to union with God but also as a limited creature dependent on the Creator. In Christ, the thematic character of the beloved does not compete with God's primacy because concern for the beloved is motivated by God and directed to God: "in loving the partner we love Christ simultaneously. *In* the beloved we love Christ."[56]

D. TRANSFORMATION OF MARRIAGE

Von Hildebrand repeatedly affirms the uniquely sublime character of sacramental marriage. He writes,

> Great as is this permanent community of love in itself, marriage objectively as well as subjectively is all the more sublime in Christ and the Holy Church. Christian marriage solemnly engaged in for Christ and in Christ, in the light of eternity, and carrying with it a sense of the deepest responsibility, differs radically from even the noblest natural marriage in which one spouse sees the other only within the limits of the natural order. A world of difference separates the two.[57]

In addition to themes related to procreation, which are discussed below, von Hildebrand's discussion of the transformation of marriage in Christ focuses on four themes: the proper motivation for marriage, the sacramental character of marriage, the indissolubility of marriage, and the three types of marriage.

In the Christian context, the fully adequate motivation for marriage involves, in addition to conjugal love, the firm belief that this association will lead both spouses to eternal salvation.[58] Marriage is a vocation, a call from God.[59] Not only can one marry and go to heaven, but God has established marriage as a particular path to lead souls to His eternal Kingdom. For the one called to marriage, God presents the beloved as a particular complement to his character.[60] The conviction that the other person is "determined by God for me and I am determined for them, that God has willed both to love one another conjugally, is the only motive that makes this community truly meaningful and desirable."[61]

Since marriage involves God's will and one's salvation, much is at stake in discerning marriage. Entering marriage involves risk. This risk, however, should not imply recklessness, but rather demonstrates the need to acknowledge marriage's seriousness: "All great decisions, insofar as they carry with them great risks, should be deeply considered before we undertake them. The conclusion of marriage calls for a full realization of the great and decisive step which it represents, and requires profound self-examination."[62]

When lovers discern whether or not they should enter marriage, they should avoid certain inadmissible motives such as "interest in economic advantages" or "the desire to participate in the worldly position of the partner or to bear his name, and to share in his influence."[63] Von Hildebrand argues that these motives are not condemned sufficiently by his fellow Catholics.[64] To encourage more authentic discernment, he offers the following:

> The precise subject of that intellectual examination should be the question as to whether the conjugal love which is here rather contemptuously treated as 'sentiment,' really exists between both persons; whether the prospective spouse is really what he seems to be; whether he is the person whom God destined for me; whether the projected union is something well pleasing to God; whether there is any danger in this union for my or his eternal welfare.[65]

The presence of authentic conjugal love, God's sanction, and the mutual eternal welfare of the lovers is the proper motivation for marriage, not mere financial gain or worldly position.

The western tradition's position that spouses, and not the priest, confer the sacrament of marriage highlights the need for authentic marriage discernment.[66] Spouses must be aware of the profound commitment they make in entering marriage. This commitment is made to the beloved and also to Christ and His Church: "The conclusion of marriage, therefore . . . does not only mean that both spouses give themselves to each other in God; they give themselves anew to Christ in the other; the sacred tie is placed in the hands of Christ, is confided to Him; the marriage bond belongs to Him."[67] Von Hildebrand even affirms that marriage entails "a consecration to God which may be likened to a religious vow."[68] Like one entering religious life, spouses entering marriage respond to God's call and express their marital vows before God and God's people.[69]

Since marriage responds to God's call, the spouses' love of one another does not compete with but rather promotes their love of God: "As the bond has been concluded in Jesus and toward Jesus, the increase of conjugal love also means a growth of the love of Jesus. The unique abandonment to the beloved opens our heart and enables it to love more and more."[70] In this sense, the spouses' actualization of conjugal love is "a *divine service*."[71] Marriage participates "directly in the establishment of the Kingdom of God."[72]

While maintaining that conjugal love flows toward love of God, von Hildebrand insists that the primary flow of love is from God to man. He begins *Marriage* by quoting Ephesians, "Husbands love your wives as Christ loved the Church."[73] He then expands these words to include a call for both husband and wife: "In marriage as a community brought to fruition in Christ and above all in marriage as a sacrament, the focus of the principle becomes the attempt to imitate the love of Christ for the Church."[74] God's love, therefore, as manifested in Christ's love of the Church, serves as an ideal for married spouses.

In addition to serving as an ideal of love, God's love also serves as an empowering source for conjugal love. Christ raised marriage to a sacrament and therefore made marriage a unique source of God's sanctifying grace.[75] These graces are particularly suited to transform spouses so that they may more authentically image in their spousal love, Christ's love for His people. These graces speak to the complementary relationship between marriage and the religious life. Whereas marriage surpasses religious life as a sacrament, religious life is superior to marriage in its intimate connection with the sacred.[76] The uniqueness of religious life lies not in the absence of marriage and conjugal love but in a surplus of love. Unlike spousal love, the love of consecrated virgins does not only point to Jesus, but "there is in virginity marriage with Jesus Himself."[77]

Von Hildebrand proposes that "In its value marriage ranks far above all other earthly communities."[78] He argues that marriage is superior because marriage is more intimately related to God's Kingdom and the supernatural destiny of the spouses and because love is more essential in marriage than in other communities.[79] As a result, he strongly rejects the contention that the nation is a community higher than the family: "These communities are believed superior only because they are numerically vaster and have a longer life than marriage. In reality they are much inferior. The most perfect state or nation cannot glorify God as much as a perfect marriage. The only decisive question always in all things—let us never forget it—is, What is for the greater glory of God?"[80] Von Hildebrand's affirmation that the family is superior to the nation is highlighted by the historical context in which he wrote his earlier works on marriage, namely, amid the emerging ideology of the Nazi Party.

Rolando Arjonillo proposes that authors, including von Hildebrand, who in the early twentieth century emphasized marriage's personal values, were in part responding to the Nazi reduction of the family to the nation.[81] This observation is especially relevant for discussion of von Hildebrand's writings since his opposition to the Nazi Party is well-documented. Von Hildebrand must have had the Nazi Party at least partially in mind when he wrote a new preface to *Marriage* in 1942:

> Our epoch is characterized by a terrible anti-personalism, a progressive blindness toward the nature and dignity of the spiritual person. This anti-personalism expresses itself mainly in a radical collectivism and in the different kinds of materialism. Of these, biological materialism is perhaps the most dangerous, for it considers man as a more highly developed animal, his whole personality determined by mere physiological elements. Human life is considered exclusively from a biological point of view and biological principles are the measure by which all human activities are judged.
>
> In such an ideological situation, it seems very important to stress again the spiritual significance of marriage—and to explain not only the primary end of procreation, but its primary meaning as the intimate union of two persons in mutual love.[82]

Marriages are not merely children factories for the nation, but a sacramental path to holiness building up the in-breaking Kingdom of God.

Commitment to Christ also transforms and solidifies marital indissolubility. All marriages have a character of stability: "marriage, even among pagans, cannot be dissolved according to the whim of the partners."[83] Nonetheless, such marriages may be dissolved if they meet the criteria of "the Pauline privilege."[84] Only consummated, sacramental marriages possess "that full validity and reality which make it absolutely indissoluble."[85]

The indissolubility of marriage is rooted in scripture. Von Hildebrand quotes the words of Jesus as written in the Gospel of Mark: "Because of the hardness of your heart he wrote you that precept. But from the beginning of the creation God made them male and female. For this cause a man shall leave his father and mother, and cleave to his wife, and the two shall become one flesh. Therefore now they are no longer two, but one flesh. What therefore God has joined together, let no man put asunder."[86] God intended marriage to be indissoluble from the beginning and Christ re-establishes this plan.[87] Marriage's indissolubility also is affirmed by Saint Paul, who describes marriage in terms of Christ's relationship with His Church. Von Hildebrand writes, "Only sacramental marriage as an image of the union of Christ and the Church possesses that full validity and reality which make it absolutely indissoluble."[88] As an image of Christ's love, spouses are called to be examples of the enduring faithfulness of Christ, who never forsakes the Church.

Marriage's indissolubility also is rooted in the intimate union shared by spouses, in their becoming "two in one flesh."[89] Von Hildebrand writes: "How superficial it is not to see the radical indissolubility of marriage as flowing from its nature as an intimate communion of love."[90] The life-long commitment of marriage has other positive consequences for the common good such as preventing "the decay of society" and safeguarding "the education of children." Nonetheless, unlike spousal union, which relates directly to marriage indissolubility, these other fruits "pertain only indirectly."[91]

Concerning the Church's struggle to uphold the indissolubility of marriage, von Hildebrand argues that few things have caused more conflicts, desertions, and apostasies: "It sometimes demands the greatest of sacrifices."[92] He explains that in extreme cases, the indissolubility of marriage may even demand remaining in an unhappy marriage when one could enter into a happy marriage.[93] Nonetheless, he argues that marriage's life-long commitment is not a hindrance to authentic love: "For the real lover, the consciousness of being indissolubly united with the beloved in Christ . . . is a source of the highest satisfaction. For he wants to become one with the beloved, and he is grateful and happy that this unity can be realized to so great a degree that it rises above all emotional changes."[94] True lovers will find the objective bond of marriage to be freeing and fulfilling.

The empowering character of marriage's indissolubility does not entail that marriage is easy for those who have authentic love. Marriage is not for the faint of heart. The one who intends to avoid all possible crosses "excludes everything that gives human life grandeur and depth. He will never know real abandon—never real, deep happiness . . . he will always provide for a possibility of retreat.[95] As a calling from God and a path to holiness, marital life includes the cross. Spouses must make sacrifices and "must fight against a weakening of [their] love."[96]

While all spouses are required to cultivate their conjugal love once they enter marriage, they are not expected to be the perfect embodiment of conjugal love. The task differs according to the distinct character of the spouses and their marriage: "God gives mankind grace in different measures, and demands more from them according to the measure of grace received."[97] Von Hildebrand discusses three levels of marriage: ultimate marriage, highest possible marriage, and marriage of renunciation.

Certain spouses are called to live marriage to the fullest. They view marriage as God's calling, as a mutual path to heaven, and as an image of Christ's love for the Church. For those spouses who contain the possibility of a profound conjugal love,

> it becomes the duty of both partners, once the marriage is concluded, to strive toward the realization of this ideal. . . . They must avoid everything that could obscure or mar this love: for instance, the absorption of the husband in his business affairs or of the wife in household duties. But above all, they must beware of an indolent indifference and of simply floating down the stream of everyday habits. They must recall anew every hour the unspeakably precious gift which God gave in the form of the soul of the beloved.[98]

In such marriages, the spouses share their lives in intimate union.

Other spouses may share an authentic love for one another, but lack the glowing character of ultimate conjugal love.[99] Their task is to attain the most profound conjugal love within the limits of possibility.[100] Such spouses should not despair when they do not embody the ideal but rather should recognize the gift of their love and do what can be done to strengthen their marital union.

Thirdly, von Hildebrand discusses those marriages in which love is completely lacking in one of the two spouses. After giving the example of Saint Monica, von Hildebrand writes,

> the obligation to live up to the objective tie which the conclusion of marriage has created persists, in spite of the fact that the combination of the two partners does not make possible the realization of ideal conjugal love. The one spouse can only love the other in a particular form of neighborly love—love him because it was with him

that the tie of marriage was knit. The task in this special case consists primarily in sacrifice and renunciation and in care for the salvation of the other.[101]

The bond of marriage remains even when one spouse does not live up to his marriage commitments. The possibility of such a relationship strongly highlights the risk of entering marriage. A marriage of renunciation differs significantly from a profound marriage or even a marriage which seeks the highest possible spousal union. Since conjugal love requires mutuality, conjugal love is undermined when one spouse is completely lacking in love. Nonetheless, the marriage bond remains.

These three categories should not embolden couples to live a life less than what they are called to in marriage. The categories, by highlighting the unique call of each marriage, are an encouragement to all spouses to further conversion. Every spouse is called to build the Kingdom of God and to promote "mutual love and conjugal faithfulness."[102]

E. SUMMARY

Von Hildebrand proposes that conjugal love is distinct from other types of love. He argues that conjugal love can exist only between a man and a woman and that this love involves a respect for the other's complete personality, making the other thematic, mutuality, intention for union, a definite decision of love, an intention for duration, a complete gift of self, and an exclusive belonging that opens one to the world. The beauty and strength of von Hildebrand's analysis is his articulation of those features uniquely characteristic of conjugal love. His discussion provides a helpful guide for discerning the presence of authentic conjugal love.

Von Hildebrand's personalist and phenomenological background are strongly evidenced in his treatment of conjugal love. He assumes that his readers have witnessed or experienced this type of love and his mode of presentation seeks to uncover the significance and meaning of this experience. He rarely quotes other authors and when he does he often employs the quotations to support what he has discussed rather than to serve as a foundation for his positions. Accordingly, the force of his argument is dependent on his ability to treat conjugal love in a manner that both is compelling and corresponds with the experience of his readers. Despite his reliance on experience, von Hildebrand's account of conjugal love clearly is indebted to the Catholic tradition. This indebtedness is revealed most clearly when he discusses natural marriage and the transformation of conjugal love and marriage that occurs in the light of Christ.

Von Hildebrand explains in detail the relationship between conjugal love and marriage. He affirms that conjugal love is the only *fully* adequate motive for marriage. Everyone seeking to enter marriage must be motivated by the foundation of conjugal love, that is, the beloved's personality as such, in order to enter marriage *morally*. Those who enter marriage with less than ideal motives are still obligated, once marriage has been established, to foster conjugal love for one another. While conjugal love anticipates marriage, marriage also requires that the spouses make a formal and solemn consent of their will. Spousal consent gives the relationship a new, objective status and gives the spouses a new responsibility to promote their conjugal love for one another.

The nature of conjugal love is not eliminated in the Christian framework but rather deepened and transfigured. Christ reveals to the lover the unique dignity of the beloved and calls the lover to seek not only the earthly good of the beloved but the beloved's eternal well-being. Further, the Christian framework reveals that conjugal love complements love of Christ.

Marriage is a vocation, that is, a calling from God which must be discerned earnestly. One ought to enter marriage because God is calling one to unite with this particular person and because God has chosen to offer His gift of salvation and grace uniquely through this person. Christ raised marriage to a sacrament, and thereby gives spouses the sanctifying grace they need to embrace the crosses of married life and to attain a life of holiness. Von Hildebrand explains the ideal of Christian marriage in relation to those many marriages that struggle to embody the high calling of marriage. He proposes that each spouse must take advantage of those opportunities available to promote conjugal love and the ideal of marriage.

Near the end of *Marriage*, von Hildebrand provides a helpful summary of his reflections on conjugal love and marriage. He describes the "grandeur and mysterious sublimity of Christian marriage" as a "most intimate communion of love in Jesus and for Jesus, which belongs to Jesus and brings about the sanctification of both spouses, in which two persons are one in one flesh and have been allowed to participate in the creation of a new human being by God, a community elevated to a sacrament as an image of the union of Christ and the Church."[103] With this summary of sacramental marriage in mind, I now turn to von Hildebrand's remarks on the consummation of marriage.

Notes

1. The work breaks down as follows: conjugal love (3-17), natural marriage (17-32), the Christians transformation of conjugal love (34-40), and sacramental marriage (40-64). The division of von Hildebrand's *Marriage* into two parts is indicated by a break in text as well as in his remarks near the beginning of the work: "Before examining the nature, the meaning and beauty of Christian marriage, which Saint Paul calls 'a great sacrament in Christ and the Holy Church,' we shall examine the essence and meaning of marriage in the realm of nature, and its specific character in reference to all other fellowships and communities" (2).

2. In German, von Hildebrand uses the term "eheliche Liebe" to describe the unique type of love between a man and a woman that is ordered toward marriage. Those who translate his works to English variously translate "eheliche Liebe" as "conjugal love," "spousal love," and "marital love." Each of these three terms are synonymous in von Hildebrand's writings since they are each translations of "eheliche Liebe." In my analysis, I have chosen to use consistently the term "conjugal love" in order to represent von Hildebrand's consistent use of "eheliche Liebe." Exceptions occur when I quote published English translations or the rare case when I use "spousal" to avoid excessive repetition of the word conjugal.

3. *The Encyclical "Humanae Vitae,"* 3; see also *Man and Woman*, 79 and 81.

4. *Marriage*, 2.

5. For more on von Hildebrand's value response morality see his *Christian Ethics* (New York: David McKay, 1953); see also Josef Seifert, "Dietrich von Hildebrands philosophische Entdeckung der 'Wertantwort' und die Grundlegung der Ethik,"*Aletheia* 5 (1992): 34-58.

6. *Marriage*, 7; see also *Man and Woman*, 16.

7. For further discussion of the concept of theme in von Hildebrand's writings, see *Christian Ethics*, 382-84.

8. *Marriage*, 8.

9. *Marriage*, 12-14.

10. *Marriage*, 9, italics in work cited.

11. Von Hildebrand writes, "Nothing is more mistaken than the adage that, 'Love is blind'" (*Marriage*, 9).

12. *Marriage*, 9, italics in work cited. In a book review of *Marriage*, John C. Ford places inordinate focus on von Hildebrand's affirmation that love can arise suddenly. Whereas von Hildebrand asserts that conjugal love *can* develop suddenly, but then gives the point limited discussion, Ford proposes that this sudden character of development is central to von Hildebrand's definition of conjugal love. Ford writes, "Can it be right to give a purported *essential* definition of conjugal love which is based, partially at least, on blind emotion and instinct?" (review of *Marriage*, by Dietrich von Hildebrand, *Thought* 17 [September 1942]: 545, italics in work cited). Ford neglects von Hildebrand's proposal that in conjugal love the lover sees the beloved's complete personality, an omission that has far reaching implications. Ford writes, "It would seem therefore that this conjugal love which is in some sense essential to marriage is partly instinctive, based on emotion, and to that extent beyond the control of the will" (544). Ford further argues that von Hildebrand "seems not to offer any criteria by which real love is to be distinguished ahead of time from infatuation" (544). On the contrary, von Hildebrand identifies a number of features distinctive to conjugal love and therefore provides helpful guidance in discerning between infatuation and conjugal love.

13. *Marriage*, 5-6.

14. *Marriage*, 6.

15. *Man and Woman*, 12.

16. *Man and Woman*, 16.

17. *Man and Woman*, 16; see also *Marriage*, 6-7 and Dietrich von Hildebrand, *Metaphysik der Gemeinschaft: Untersuchungen über Wesen und Wert der Gemeinschaft*, vol. 4 of *Dietrich von Hildebrand Gesammelte Werke*, ed. Dietrich von Hildebrand Gesellschaft (Regensburg: Josef Habbel, 1975), 35-36, 234-39, and 306.

18. *Marriage*, 7, italics in work cited.

19. *The Encyclical "Humanae Vitae,"* 5.

20. *Marriage*, 10.

21. *Marriage*, 10, 11-12. Von Hildebrand does not explain the basis on which he makes this claim. He simply states the observation and moves on. For further discussion of the difference between man and woman and the complementary character of those differences, see Dietrich von Hildebrand, *Man and Woman* (Chicago, IL: Franciscan Herald Press, 1966), 58-66.

22. *The Encyclical "Humanae Vitae,"* 16.

23. *Marriage*, 15.

24. *Marriage*, 15.

25. When von Hildebrand discusses the proper motivations for marriage, he notes the need to test conjugal love (*Marriage*, 56). This will be discussed further below.

26. *Marriage*, 8.
27. *Marriage*, 14.
28. *Marriage*, 14; see also 49.
29. *Marriage*, 5; see also 7, 12, and 15.
30. *Marriage*, 60.
31. *Marriage*, 16. Note the difference between von Hildebrand's treatment of polygamy in his work, *Marriage*, and Augustine's defense of Abraham's polygamy found near the end of his work, *On the Good of Marriage*. Concerning the polygamy of the Old Testament Patriarchs, Augustine writes, "that is no sin, which is committed neither against nature, in that they used those women not for wantonness, but for the begetting of children: nor against custom, forasmuch as such things were usually done at those times: nor against command, forasmuch as they were forbidden by no law" (Augustine, *On the Good of Marriage*, trans. C. L. Cornish, in *Nicene and Post-Nicene Fathers*, vol. 3, ed. Philip Schaff [Peabody, MA: Hendrickson, 1994], section 33, 413). Von Hildebrand argues that conjugal love excludes polygamy even prior to the marriage contract. The distinction between the two authors seems to lie in Augustine's respect for Abraham and von Hildebrand's attentiveness to both the inter-personal values of marriage and the dignity of women. Augustine writes near the beginning of *On the Good of Marriage* that man and woman can have "a certain friendly and true union of the one ruling, and the other obeying" (p. 399; see also 405 where he refers to women as being weaker than men).
32. *Marriage*, 17.
33. *Marriage*, 13, italics and capitalization of ego in work cited. See also *Man and Woman*, 64, where von Hildebrand describes these same effects in terms of the "spiritual fecundation" that generally results from man's spiritual contact with woman.
34. *Marriage*, 17.
35. *The Encyclical "Humanae Vitae,"* 6, 20-21; see also *Man and Woman*, 80.
36. *Marriage*, 54. The first sentence of this quote suggests that while being motivated by love would be ideal, one morally could enter marriage without love for another. Such a conclusion, however, does not correspond with what von Hildebrand argues elsewhere and with what von Hildebrand wrote in the original German. The words "Although love" at the beginning of the quoted sentence are a translation of *Wenn dies*. The *dies* ("this") refers to the previous sentence in which von Hildebrand proposes that marriage is the fulfillment of *conjugal* love. What is translated as "Although love" should read "Although conjugal love." Therefore, von Hildebrand is not proposing that motives lacking *love* are morally acceptable, but making the smaller claim that entering marriage without viewing marriage as *the fulfillment of one's conjugal love* can be morally acceptable. This reading is supported by the emphasis that von Hildebrand places on the distinctiveness of conjugal love among other loves as well as the comparison, which he draws at the end of the quotation, between those who are "blunt" and those who are capable of an "ultimate conjugal love."
37. *Marriage*, 55.
38. *Marriage*, 54-55.
39. *Marriage*, 57-58, italics in original; see also 55 and *Man and Woman*, 27.
40. *Die Ehe*, 38, my translation. The German reads as follows, "Wenn auch die einmal geschlossene Ehe Liebe fordert von beiden Ehegatten, wie wir früher sahen, und die Tatsache, daß der andere der Ehemann ist oder die Ehefrau, auch ein Motiv für die Liebe darstellt." I use my own translation because the published English translation is not as clear in communicating that love is a demand of marriage. The translation instead reads as follows: "Although as we have seen, the married couple have a motive for love in the fact that they are conjugally united" (*Marriage*, 53).
41. *Marriage*, 53.
42. *Marriage*, 17; see also 18-19; *Man and Woman*, 81; and "Lambeth-Botschaft," 21.
43. "Lambeth-Botschaft," 23: "In addition, marriage, according to the Catholic conception, is not only the highest natural community of love with the end of procreation, but also an objective unity of two persons. . . . In order to understand this, one must understand generally the creative power of certain acts, which when performed originate objective products, which once originated cannot simply be resolved again" (my translation). The original German runs

as follows: "Die Ehe ist ferner nach katholischer Auffassung nicht nur die höchste natürliche Liebesgemeinschaft mit dem Zweck der Fortpflanzung, sondern auch eine objektive Einheit zweier Personen. . . . Um dies zu verstehen, muß man generell die schöpferische Kraft gewisser Akte verstehen, durch dehen Vollzug objektive Gebilde entstehen, die einmal entstanden, nicht einfach wieder aufgelöst werden können."

44. *Marriage*, 18, italics in work cited; see also 19.

45. *Marriage*, 18-19. Von Hildebrand's discussion of marriage's objective bond of marriage seems more a manifestation of Catholic commitments than a philosophical account of the objective bond of marriage.

46. *Marriage*, 27; see also 28.

47. *Marriage*, 18; see also 19.

48. *Marriage*, 21.

49. *Man and Woman*, 83.

50. Von Hildebrand writes, "The supernatural does not dissolve this finest earthly good" (*Marriage*, 34).

51. *Marriage*, 35.

52. *Marriage*, 36-37.

53. *Marriage*, 37-38; see also 38-39.

54. *Marriage*, 38; see also 60.

55. *Marriage*, 38; see also 63.

56. *Marriage*, 37, italics in work cited; see also 62.

57. *Marriage*, 34; see also 18-19 and 40-41.

58. Marriage, 53. Von Hildebrand's position differs from that of Augustine who argues that the only authentic motive for marriage is the begetting of children (*On the Good of Marriage*, trans. C. L. Cornish, in *Nicene and Post-Nicene Fathers*, vol. 3, ed. Philip Schaff [Peabody, MA: Hendrickson, 1994], 402, 403, 407, 408, and 412).

59. *Marriage*, 43-44.

60. *Marriage*, 10 and 54.

61. *Die Ehe*, 38, my translation. The German reads as follows: "daß die andere Person der für mich von Gott Bestimmte ist und ich der für sie Bestimmte, daß Gott beide in jener ehelichen Liebe verbunden hat, das Motiv, das diese Gemeinschaft allein wahrhaft sinnvoll und wünschenswert macht." The published translation states that the motives for marriage just described are the only motives "which can make this community desirable and give it meaning" (*Marriage*, 53). By not translating "wahrhaft" the translation indicates that without these motives marriage is devoid of meaning. Such a conclusion would contradict the first half of von Hildebrand's work which dealt with conjugal love and natural marriage.

62. *Marriage*, 52: see also 50.

63. *Marriage*, 55.

64. *Marriage*, 56.

65. *Marriage*, 56-57.

66. *Marriage*, 44-45; von Hildebrand contends that the spouses' role in conferring the sacrament affirms the centrality of conjugal love in marriage (*Marriage*, 45).

67. *Marriage*, 41.

68. *Marriage*, 41.

69. Von Hildebrand goes on to affirm the unique consecration offered in religious life (*Marriage*, 41).

70. *Marriage*, 62-63.

71. *Marriage*, 43, italics in work cited; see also 41.

72. *Marriage*, 1.

73. *Marriage*, 1. The quote comes from Ephesians 5:25; von Hildebrand does not indicate the translation he uses.

74. *Marriage*, 60; see also 1. In addition, von Hildebrand proposes that marriage images the final end of man, namely, eternal union with God. He writes, "What beauty is possessed by this tie, a bond which requires of us this conjugal love and implies a task which is an image of our eternal end—the union of the soul with God" (*Marriage*, 62; see also 2-3, 32, and *The Encyclical "Humanae Vitae,"* 4-5).

75. *Marriage*, 1 and 43; see also *The Encyclical "Humanae Vitae,"* 24.

76. *Marriage*, 43-44. Von Hildebrand explains that the superiority of marriage lies not in celibacy as such, but only when virginity is "chosen for the reign of God and consecrated to God" (*Marriage*, 63-64; see also von Hildebrand's discussion of virginity in *Purity*, 87-142).

77. *Marriage*, 63.

78. *Marriage*, 58.

79. *Marriage*, 58-59; see also 61 where von Hildebrand proposes that insofar as spouses are uniquely concerned for one another, "marriage is also more free of egoism" than other communities.

80. *Marriage*, 60-61; see also 59 where von Hildebrand writes, "A community infinitely higher than the nation is the family."

81. Rolando B. Arjonillo, *Conjugal Love of the Ends of Marriage: A Study of Dietrich von Hildebrand and Herbert Doms in the Light of the Pastoral Constitution "Gaudium et Spes"* (Bern: Lang, 1998), 31; for more on family policy in Germany from 1918-1945, see Michelle Mouton, *From Nurturing the Nation to Purifying the Volk: Weimar and Nazi Family Policy, 1918-1945* (New York: Cambridge University Press, 2007).

82. *Marriage*, v.

83. *Marriage*, 46. He affirms that "the indissolubility of sacramental marriage is not merely the result of a positive law of God" separate from "the nature of marriage" (*Marriage*, 46).

84. *Marriage*, 46. Von Hildebrand would have been working with the 1917 Code which describes the Pauline privilege as follows: "Legitimate marriage between the non-baptized, even if it is consummated, is dissolved in favor of the faith by the Pauline privilege" (*The 1917 Pio-Benedictine Code of Canon Law*, trans. Edward N. Peters [San Francisco, CA: Ignatius Press, 2001], canon 1120, §1; see also canon 1143 of the 1983 Code, *Code of Canon Law, Latin-English Translation: New English Translation*, trans. Canon Law Society of America [Washington, D.C.: Canon Law Society of America, 1999]). This principle is based on Paul's words to the First Corinthians: "If any brother has a wife who is an unbeliever, and she is willing to go on living with him, he should not divorce her; and if any woman has a husband who is an unbeliever, and he is willing to go on living with her, she should not divorce her husband. . . . If the unbeliever separates, however, let him separate. The brother or sister is not bound in such cases; God has called you to peace" (1 Cor. 7:12-13, 15-16). Accordingly, the Pauline privilege further requires the baptized party to establish, if possible, that the non-baptized party refuses both to be baptized and to live in peace with the baptized party (*Pio-Benedictine Code*, canons 1121-1125; see also canons 1143-1147 of the 1983 Code, *Code of Canon Law*).

85. *Marriage*, 46. Here, I emphasize the difference between natural marriage and sacramental marriage concerning indissolubility. In the next chapter, I discuss the significance of consummation in completing marriage and therefore rendering the spousal union indissoluble.

86. *The Encyclical "Humanae Vitae,"* 23, quotation of Mk. 10:5-9; von Hildebrand does not indicate the translation he employs.

87. *Marriage*, 47.

88. *Marriage*, 46; see also 33, where von Hildebrand opens the section on sacramental marriage by quoting Eph. 5:31-32: "For this cause shall a man leave his father and mother: and shall cleave to his wife, and they shall be two in one flesh. This is a great sacrament; but I speak in Christ and in the Church."

89. Von Hildebrand quotes this phrase as found in 1 Cor. 6:16 (*Marriage*, 26), as found in Eph. 5:31 (*Marriage*, 33), and as found in Mk. 10:5-9 (*The Encyclical "Humanae Vitae,"* 23; see also *Marriage*, 16 and 21), which in turn references Gen. 2:24 (*The Encyclical "Humanae Vitae,"* 23).

90. *Marriage*, 47.

91. *Marriage*, 47-48.

92. *Marriage*, 47.

93. *Marriage*, 47.

94. *Marriage*, 49, italics in work cited; see also 49-50.

95. *Marriage*, 51.

96. *Marriage*, 28.

97. *Marriage*, 29; see also 31.
98. *Marriage*, 29.
99. Von Hildebrand neither affirms nor denies that spouses can move from one category to another. The role of the three levels of marriage seem to serve von Hildebrand's affirmation that "The particular, divinely appointed meaning of an individual marriage has to be found elsewhere, inasmuch as the task varies according to what appears as the highest attainable possibility in a given combination of two characters" (*Marriage*, 31).
100. *Marriage*, 30.
101. *Marriage*, 30-31.
102. *Marriage*, 31.
103. *Marriage*, 52.

Chapter Two

The Depth of the Conjugal Act

Although von Hildebrand wrote *Purity* a few years before *Marriage*, he proposed that sex is fully understood only in the marriage context. Central to von Hildebrand's discussion of the conjugal act is his argument that sex is essentially deep.[1] In particular, he highlights the action's depth both as the consummation of marriage and as the actualization of conjugal love.

A. CONSUMMATION OF MARRIAGE

Von Hildebrand maintains that the conjugal act is not simply an expression of marriage but also a fulfillment and completion of the wedding vows.[2] This new fulfillment of marriage is manifested in the way consummation establishes the life-long bond of marriage: "The character of indissolubility begins with the consummation of the marriage, with the fully accomplished self-donation, whereby 'they shall be two in one flesh.'"[3] While von Hildebrand's remarks support the canonical function that consummation has in rendering marriage indissoluble, he affirms that this legal obligation is rooted in the nature of the conjugal act.[4] He writes, "The physical union of husband and wife constitutes such an ultimate intimacy between two human beings that of its essence it is a surrender valid once and for all."[5]

From conjugal love to consummated, sacramental marriage, one witnesses different levels of permanence. First, conjugal love itself implies that one intends a life-long union with the beloved. Yet, prior to the marriage bond, conjugal love is in the stage of discernment. Natural marriage, according to von Hildebrand, is like legislation promulgated by an appropriate authority. Such a marriage is not merely in a stage of discernment but entails an objective bond that goes beyond one's transitory dispositions. Still, in unique circumstances, the Pauline privilege allows for the dissolution of non-sacramental marriages where the good faith of at least one party calls for the dissolution.[6] Sacramental marriage, that is, a marriage ratified when two baptized spouses declare their wedding vows, is a life-long union not subject to the Pauline privilege. Nonetheless, even here, the union can be dissolved by the Apostolic See in unique situations when the marriage is not consummated.[7] Finally, a ratified and consummated marriage between two baptized Christians is absolutely indissoluble. In such cases, "What God has joined together, no human being must separate" (Mt. 19:6).[8]

Von Hildebrand proposes that the conjugal act should be expressed only with God's sanction.[9] God grants this approval only in the context of marriage: "Man must feel for sex [the sexual sphere] an awe which no other sphere demands—an awe which permits his access only if God in a special fashion should give him leave, as He gives it in the *sacrament* of matrimony."[10] Von Hildebrand is not proposing that *married* couples can express the conjugal act at any time or in any manner and be assured of God's approval. Marriage is necessary but not sufficient for God's sanction. Even married spouses must further discern when and in what manner the conjugal act ought to be expressed.[11]

Von Hildebrand's use of the term "conjugal love" may give the impression that he opens the door for expression of sexual union outside of marriage. He uses "conjugal love" to describe both the love of couples before marriage and love committed in marriage. Therefore, when he affirms that the conjugal act is an actualization of conjugal love, one must note that he means conjugal love committed in marriage.[12] Von Hildebrand critiques those who seek to eliminate the "taboo" of extramarital intercourse:

> These people believe that in neutralizing sex from the moral point of view, they finally approach it in a positive way. But in reality, the moral significance of this sphere is indissolubly linked with its true nature, with its true value, with the mystery it embodies. And in trying to draw sex out of the moral universe, they do not open the way for a healthy approach to sex. They make man blind to its true value; they bar the stream of deep happiness which it is destined to bestow on human life in marriage. Instead of freeing man, they imprison him in hopeless boredom.[13]

The conjugal act is a noble action that completes the sacrament of marriage and the failure to respect the action's nobility is a desecration of both conjugal love and marriage.[14]

B. ACTUALIZATION OF CONJUGAL LOVE

Since conjugal love is the authentic motivation for and an obligation of marriage, and since the conjugal act is the completion and fulfillment of marriage, von Hildebrand's affirmation that the sexual sphere is intimately connected with conjugal love simply connects the dots:

> Between it [the sexual sphere] and wedded love there subsists a pre-established harmony. Its true significance as an experience is inseparable from its character as the expression and flower of a specific kind of love. The man who has grasped the meaning of sex [the sexual sphere] recognizes . . . the unique connection which subsists between physical sex [the sexual sphere] and wedded love.[15]

One can understand the conjugal act only from the higher and more fundamental reality of conjugal love.[16] The conjugal act is "the specific expression and fulfilment of wedded love and its longing for fuller communion."[17]

One manner in which spouses actualize their conjugal love in the marital act is the distinctive way in which they give themselves to one another.[18] This unique type of giving involves "a *surrender* of one's self to the other."[19] The foundation of the unique self-gift actualized in the conjugal act is the intimate place the sexual sphere holds in man's personality: "In a certain sense sex [the sexual sphere] is the secret of the individual. . . . It is something which the person concerned feels to be altogether private, something which belongs to his inmost being."[20] When one expresses one's sexuality one reveals something central to one's personality: "It is the initiation of another into our secret. . . . And because sex is the secret of the individual, to disclose and surrender it is in a unique sense to surrender oneself."[21]

Von Hildebrand argues that the conjugal act's self-revelatory character is affirmed in the Scriptures, which refer to the conjugal act as a "knowing" of one's spouse: "It is a very significant and deep fact that the Bible speaks of this bodily union as a 'knowing'; to know a woman. This term expresses the intimacy and depth of the disclosure of the secret of the person, the self-donation which this union embodies."[22]

The deep revelation of the person found in the conjugal act is manifested in the sexual sphere's bodily appetite. The sexual appetite has a depth that other appetites, such as eating, drinking, and sleeping, only approach when pushed against the necessities of life.[23] Since the sexual sphere deals with the person's intimate secret and since sexual desire is strong, one must work to refrain from a shallow expression of sex. This is in part accomplished through attentiveness to the experience of shame.

Shame can be distinguished into two categories. The first type of shame can make "a man seek to hide any personal ugliness or deformity"; it is "the shame which tries to conceal a fault."[24] The characteristic feature of this shame "is the fear of appearing ludicrous."[25]

The second type of shame is an "incomparably deeper and thoroughly noble shame which conceals something because it is particularly intimate; for example, when a man is ashamed to show his most delicate and deepest feelings to outsiders."[26] Concerning this second type of shame as it relates to the sexual sphere, von Hildebrand writes that "to misinterpret this bashfulness and modesty, which is called for in the sphere of sex, as mere prudery, is to exhibit the same deplorable blindness and superficiality which confuses humility with servility, and purity with frigidity."[27] The experience of shame, then, does not necessarily entail the concealing of something ugly but can involve the protection of something both intimate and noble.[28]

Accordingly, von Hildebrand spends a significant amount of time distinguishing between the proper expression of one's sexuality and the temperament of insensuality. He explains that the term sensuous can be applied to a man who has an inclination toward sexual things but most often is used to describe a man who tends to have powerful desires.[29] Insensuousness, then, can mean one of three things: the absence of strong instincts, a lack in understanding sex's peculiarity, or a lack of susceptibility to sex.[30]

Von Hildebrand adamantly opposes the argument that one must be insensuous to express properly one's sexuality. He writes, "the absence of a sexual temperament in no way connotes a particularly high degree of spirituality, any more than, *mutatis mutandis*, actual poverty connotes an interior independence of possessions."[31] He paints a rather unfavorable picture of the man who sees insensuousness as the ideal:

> We often come across men who will to be pure, who, wherever they recognise its [the sexual sphere's] presence, carefully avoid any conscious surrender to sex [the sexual sphere] taken in isolation for its own sake, but who nevertheless are not genuinely pure, for they seek and find a certain sexual [sensual] satisfaction in their love of excitement, their craving to make an impression, their sensibility, their self-importance, their carriage, the entire rhythm, of their lives. Men of this type often consider themselves particularly pure, and speak of sex [the sexual sphere] with disgust. They consider themselves raised far above everything sexual, even perhaps despise the union of wedlock, because they consider it too fleshly and themselves too precious to surrender their person to another in this fashion.[32]

Sensuousness is not a moral disposition but simply a temperament.[33]

The appropriate moral disposition toward the sexual sphere is not one that denies the sphere's value, but rather one that understands this value and thereby understands how the sexual sphere is to be adequately expressed. In this regard, insensuousness is not even favorable to purity.[34] The crucial moral tension, for one's expression of the conjugal act, is not between sexual desire and the will's refusal to give into that desire, but discerning when one consciously can express the conjugal act so freely and actively that the action takes up sexual desire and directs that desire in a noble manner.[35]

Only when the conjugal act is understood as an expression of conjugal love committed in marriage, an affirmation of the beloved, and a mutual self-giving does the intense desire of the sexual sphere become intelligible. Von Hildebrand writes, "For the joy and attraction are here the result of the unique union, the mutual contact in the sexual sphere, the most intimate mutual self-donation and self-revelation, and, moreover, the consciousness of a union willed by God—all factors that are operative only when sex is exercised on the basis of wedded love."[36]

The conjugal act further actualizes conjugal love as the fulfillment of the spouses' desired union: "And just because sex [the sexual sphere] is so uniquely intimate and represents the secret of the person concerned, the sexual gift of one person to another signifies an incomparably close union with that other and a self-surrender to him or her."[37] Von Hildebrand argues that an orientation toward unity is an essential characteristic of the sexual sphere: "We cannot grasp the mystery embodied in this sphere until we grasp that its deepest meaning consists in being a unique fulfillment of spousal love and its desire for union."[38]

The conjugal act is the highest, most intimate expression of union among human persons.[39] Von Hildebrand describes sexual union with the biblical imagery of the two becoming one flesh.[40] Nonetheless, the conjugal act does not entail a literal, spiritual and bodily fusion of two persons, a position von Hildebrand maintains is "absurd if not impossible."[41] The conjugal act need not be a literal union to be intimate. The spousal desire for union characteristic of conjugal love and uniquely actualized in the conjugal act are key themes in von Hildebrand's account of the conjugal act. He argues that this spousal union has unique value as an image of the heavenly union between God and the human soul.[42]

The conjugal act's role in consummating marriage and actualizing conjugal love demonstrates the always significant character of the conjugal act.[43] A further manifestation of this action's depth is the manner in which the action forms one's personality.[44] Von Hildebrand explains that the conjugal act is related to a number of moral virtues. In addition to the connection between the conjugal act and the virtue of wedded love, von Hildebrand affirms that one's disposition toward the conjugal act and the sexual sphere is uniquely related to the virtue of purity. He writes, "According to the attitude which a man adopts to sex [the sexual sphere] he is pure or impure."[45] Since one's sexuality is central to man, von Hildebrand explains that purity's development is integral to human flourishing. He writes, "The sexually insensible is as such an incomplete man, to whom a very profound zone of human nature is closed. . . . The pure man, on the contrary, is the only man who is truly complete. In him a central orientation of human nature is fulfilled, and everything which the sexually insensible lacked he possesses in its entirety."[46]

Other virtues that von Hildebrand discusses in relation to the sexual sphere include reverence,[47] modesty,[48] chastity,[49] respect,[50] warmheartedness,[51] humility,[52] gentleness,[53] and peace.[54] Moreover, von Hildebrand discusses the fulfillment of freedom that occurs when the conjugal act is a God-sanctioned expression and fulfillment of conjugal love. He writes, "When sex is thus experienced there is no seduction in it, but liberation, pathos, and solemn earnest."[55]

C. MISUSES OF THE CONJUGAL ACT

The depth of sexual union means that it can be either a profound actualization or desecration of the sacrament of marriage and conjugal love. Von Hildebrand explains that "precisely because of this nobility and sacred mystery, because of the great value which it is destined to realize, every abuse is a terrible sin, and even contains something sacrilegious."[56] The depth of sexual desire manifests the nobility of the sexual sphere but also can tempt one to misuse the conjugal act. Von Hildebrand writes, "It is the tragedy of fallen man that the *danger* at least of this perversion is always present, the danger that sex [the sexual sphere] should exercise over him this baser appeal."[57] Von Hildebrand discusses three misuses of the conjugal act: a giving into seductive charm, a failure to perceive the peculiarity of sex, and diabolic lust.[58]

Central to von Hildebrand's discussion of the sexual sphere's seductive charm is his use of the term "vital-corporeality." Although he does not define "vital-corporeality" in *Purity,* the term appears to have a similar meaning as "animal voluntariness," a concept he articulates in *Christian Ethics*. Animal action has a certain voluntariness expressed when an animal decides between different instincts or natural tendencies. This partiality is not freedom in the truest sense because the choice is merely the result of internal instincts and external causes.[59] Man too has internal instincts and these forces can lead to action without the sanction of human freedom. This is the threat posed by the power of vital-corporeality.

The first danger of the sexual act is the threat that sex's vital-corporeality will overwhelm one's spirit: "The orgasm in its violence, its fury, its convulsion, has a tendency to overpower the spirit."[60] Unlike animals, man has a spiritual realm which ought to govern the vital corporeal. This spiritual realm has the capacity to understand the importance of the objects before him, and is the center from which he freely chooses to give due response to these objects. Man's spiritual dimension gives action personal vitality so that when the spirit is overthrown, action in a sense is rendered sterile.[61]

Von Hildebrand writes that "a moral absorption is always involved in the sexual act, unless the spirit is at the same time brought into action in a fashion correspondingly profound."[62] The lover and the beloved must make sure they are prepared to authentically give themselves to one another in the conjugal act. The spouses must express this action freely and consciously: "Any breath of levity, any even momentary self-forgetfulness under the influence of passion, any abandonment to the passing moment, contradicts radically the significance of this union, its ultimacy, its seriousness and its irrevocability, and therefore always involves not only objectively, but *subjectively* also, a material impurity; indeed, in a certain sense, a desecration."[63] If the spouses fail to have this consciousness in their expression of the conjugal act, they are susceptible to being dragged by their vital-corporeality. Von Hildebrand argues that to lose control of one's self in this way is an improper response "to the very nature and value of the sphere of sex."[64]

Von Hildebrand distinguishes between giving one's self to the beloved in the conjugal act and losing one's self to sexual desire.[65] The lover's surrender to his spouse ought to be discerned and should be given both freely and consciously. Surrender in this sense refers to the intensity of the self-gift offered by the lover. The lover uniquely gives his life to the beloved so that the lover is said to belong to the beloved. In contrast, one's surrender to sexual desire is not a free giving of one's self but a losing of one's self to the strong drive of the sexual sphere.[66]

In the second misuse of the conjugal act, typified by what von Hildebrand refers to as the fleshly disposition, the moral agent does not give into vital corporeality, but fails to recognize the conjugal act's depth altogether.[67] The fleshly "abuse sex [the sexual sphere], not by perverting its distinctive quality to evil, but because they utterly fail to perceive it; . . . like the animals, they 'make use' of sex [this sphere]."[68] Such men do not realize that the conjugal act is intended to be the actualization of a deep love because they view the conjugal act simply as the satisfaction of sexual instinct.[69]

Von Hildebrand maintains that this second misuse of the conjugal act goes further astray than the first:

> The one who falls morally but is aware of his immorality remains still in the orbit of truth; he acknowledges the ultimate importance of the moral question, even if he goes astray in this moment. He still moves in the true spiritual universe and sees the true values. His situation may be tragic. Whereas the one who desecrates the mystery of sex by seeing in it a harmless satisfaction of a bodily instinct . . . is not tragic, but he is immersed in hopeless boredom; because it is the moral light, the great tension of good and evil, which elevates and widens human life beyond the frontiers of our earthly existence.[70]

Von Hildebrand argues that one's recognition of the sexual sphere's value is presupposed for fruitful discussion of sexual ethics.[71] He further proposes that ignorance of the sexual sphere is the unique problem of his time: "What I deplore in the approach to sex today is not primarily the immorality—which was equally to be found in former times—but the widespread blindness toward the very nature and meaning of this sphere."[72]

The isolation of sexual pleasure, however, according to von Hildebrand, is particularly harmful.[73] He refers to such a disposition as a diabolic evil lust.[74] This position differs from the second misuse because whereas the fleshly man fails to act morally because of his ignorance of the sexual sphere's depth, the man with a diabolic lust denies the values of conjugal love, marriage, and the participating person.[75]

When one misuses the conjugal act, the action maintains a central place in personal formation. However, the misuse works not toward virtue but in the opposite direction toward degradation, defilement, desecration, and the inability to express the conjugal act. Von Hildebrand argues that the misuse of sex degrades all persons involved: "Where the foundation has not been laid by wedded love and the deliberate purpose of forming a permanent objective community of life, secure from arbitrary whim, the act, which represents a unique self-donation and effects an intimate union of the most fundamental nature, signifies a specific squandering of self, the betrayal of one's self and one's partner."[76] Since the conjugal act reveals the person's intimate secret, the shallow expression of the act degrades those involved by indicating that they have little value.

Von Hildebrand further argues that the "abuse of sex always involves a second factor, a *desecration*."[77] He affirms that desecration in general is when one employs "something destined for a sublime purpose in a fashion inconsistent with that noble object—as for instance to utter God's Name thoughtlessly or irreverently."[78] In the case of the conjugal act, the spouses are related to a number of noble objects: the dignity of the human person, the Sacrament of marriage, and the depth of the conjugal act. Von Hildebrand writes,

> To perform the act which signifies the hallowed union of two human beings in one flesh and should be the expression and fulfillment of a lasting and indissoluble bond of love—and which effects the most perfect self-surrender to another, because it involves the mutual revelation of a secret, a self-revelation, that is to say, of the most intimate character, with a partner to whom we are not united by the sacred tie of matrimony is obviously a desecration of the most awful kind.[79]

A desecration results both when one abuses the conjugal act and when one expresses the action in a fashion that fails to manifest the conjugal act's lofty purpose.[80]

Von Hildebrand proposes that the abuse of sex "further involves a specific defilement"[81] This defilement involves first a unique fleshly bondage of the spirit: "the 'sensualisation' of the spirit which results from surrender to this pleasure differs not only in degree, but in quality, from the entirely different 'sensualisation' to which the glutton exposes himself."[82] This defilement further involves an apostasy from God. Since man must employ his spiritual powers to stand in right relationship with God, the one who surrenders his spirit to sexual desire "separates himself in an altogether unique fashion from God."[83] The personal defilement resulting from the sexual sphere's misuse "stands in peculiar contrast to the sphere of holiness, the home of liberation and sublimation, resplendent with the light of peace. And it further involves a specific opposition to the peculiar quality of expansive warmheartedness which belongs to pure love as such."[84]

Von Hildebrand indicates that the misuse of sex may incapacitate one's ability to express the action in an authentic manner. He argues, "To approach sex as a mere instinct like hunger and thirst destroys the possibility of the great and deep experience of the bodily union."[85] However, this incapacitation need not have the final word. Von Hildebrand maintains that one later may have a conversion enabling him to genuinely express the conjugal act.[86] He explains the conditions necessary for such a conversion.

An act of the will does not suffice in itself for conversion. The will can diagnose the temptations in the sexual sphere and avoid giving into those temptations so that "the good intention, not to be 'swamped,' or swallowed up, is thus by itself able to exclude all moral fault when the act of wedded union is a duty."[87] However, such an act of the will does not transform disordered sexual desire but simply "overleaps" the desire or renders the disordered tendencies "to a certain point harmless."[88] He continues, "no actual transformation is thereby effected to turn the casting away of self by a change of quality into an actual self-surrender, and really transform sex as an experience, for it is this aspect which in this connection is of decisive importance."[89] Such a transformation requires wedded love.

Von Hildebrand writes that love "does not therefore act as a force which remains outside the physical event and conquers it from without, as when, for instance, a man remains spiritually untouched by severe bodily pain, but makes the physical event an expression of itself."[90] The one who has love does not fling himself away in the conjugal act or even merely prevent such a loss of self but offers himself in an authentic self-gift: "By its operation the factor of complete self-abandonment objectively contained in the orgasm is totally changed; remoulded, so to speak, from a casting away of self into a self-surrender whereby the sexual act really becomes throughout a fulfilment of wedded love's *intentio unitiva*."[91]

The conjugal act's transformation in love is performed only when the spouses stand in right relationship with God: "Only when the person remains in God, affirming his adherence to God by an explicit act, does the supreme surrender to a creature not involve 'letting oneself go.'"[92] Without having right relationship with God, the lover's surrender to the beloved risks becoming "a casting away of self of a far deeper nature [than one's surrender to sexual desire]."[93] He writes, "It is to God alone that we may, in the full sense, surrender ourselves without reserve or can do so without losing ourselves."[94] However, he further explains that in God, "man may surrender himself even to a fellow creature" insofar as this surrender is "really incorporated into the surrender to God" and is "intrinsically 'formed' by the latter."[95]

Von Hildebrand's discussion of sexual desire's transformation in marriage leads to an important qualification of marriage's *remedia concupiscentia*. He explains that this remedy is not the necessary consequence of marriage as if couples were immediately freed from sexual temptation after validly concluding marriage.[96] Rather, marriage is necessary but not sufficient for the transformation of sexual desire. The remedy of concupiscence further involves right relationship with God and commitment to spousal love: "it is the reverent knowledge that it is by God's express permission that we have crossed the frontiers of sex, which gives the soul that humble freedom, that conscious emancipation, by which we accept the fact of sex as it is, and ennoble it by the penetrating vision of love, undisturbed by the fact that here too the results of the Fall make themselves felt. . . . 'Love covereth a multitude of sins.'"[97]

D. SUMMARY

Von Hildebrand maintains that the conjugal act is necessarily deep because God intends the action to be the consummation of marriage and the actualization of spousal love. As the consummation of marriage, the conjugal act renders sacramental marriage indissoluble. For this reason, von Hildebrand maintains that the action requires God's sanction and should not be expressed prior to the marriage commitment.

As the actualization of conjugal love, the conjugal act involves a unique gift of self in which one reveals one's intimate secret to the beloved. The depth of this self-revelation is manifested in the strength of sexual desire and in the experience of shame. Shame ought to be felt not because sexual desire is evil but in order to avoid the revelation of one's person in a context where one's value is not understood or respected. The conjugal act should be a unique mutual expression of conjugal love that actualizes an intimate spousal union and fosters virtues such as reverence, modesty, and humility.

The conjugal act's depth is manifested not only as the consummation of marriage and actualization of conjugal love but also as grave misuse. Unless the spouses consciously are prepared to express the depth of the action, they risk losing their freedom to the sexual sphere's vital corporeality, that is, the strong physical dynamism of sexual union. Other misuses of the conjugal act include the failure to perceive the conjugal act's depth and the diabolic isolation of sexual pleasure.

The conjugal act's misuse leads to the degradation of persons, the desecration of marriage, a unique separation from God, and an inability to express the conjugal act. These negative consequences, however, need not have the last word. Individuals can seek conversion through acts of the will, commitment to wedded love, and right relationship with God.

A further reason the conjugal act is essentially deep is the link between the action and procreation.[98] In order to discuss that link, I now turn to von Hildebrand's central distinction between the primary meaning and the primary end of marriage. I do so only after bringing together von Hildebrand's remarks on the relationship between conjugal love, marriage, and the conjugal act. For as von Hildebrand writes, "It is possible to gauge in its fullness and depth the sublimity of the connection between sex and the origin of a new human being, or to recognize all that is implied by the fact that it is no mere living thing, but a man, who comes into existence, only if we already understand the peculiar relationship which subsists between physical sex and wedded love."[99]

Notes

1. See, for example, *Purity*, 16, where von Hildebrand writes, "Sex [the sexual sphere] is always extraordinary, but its characteristic extraordinariness assumes diametrically opposite forms. At one time it is awe-inspiring, mysterious, noble, chaste, and free; at another, illegitimate, intoxicating and befogging" (brackets my own); see also *Purity*, 5. As is the case in the above quotation, the anonymous translator of von Hildebrand's *Purity* consistently translates *die sinnliche Sphäre* as "physical sex" or "sex." A literal translation of the phrase is "the sensual sphere." The inadequacy of "physical sex" or "sex" as a translation is evident in chapter two of *Purity* where the translator leaves *sinnlich* untranslated and notes in a footnote that "sex" does not accurately translate *die sinnliche Sphäre*. Since von Hildebrand distinguishes between *die sinnliche Sphäre* (the sensual *sphere*) and *die eheliche Akt* (the marriage act), I regret that the translator often drops the word sphere in his translation of *die sinnliche Sphäre*. Although the sexual sphere finds authentic expression and fulfillment in the conjugal act, the sphere itself is not the conjugal act. Nonetheless, the translator is somewhat justified in his confusion; one cannot translate von Hildebrand's use of *sinnlich* in *Purity* with any one English term. In this regard, the translator's struggle to translate *sinnlich* anticipates a development in von Hildebrand's own use of the term. While von Hildebrand often uses *sinnlich* in his early works, *Reinheit und Jungfräulichkeit* and *Die Ehe*, when he collaborates in the 1942 English translation of *Die Ehe*, the term *sinnlich* is translated variously as "sensual" and "sexual." Von Hildebrand continues this distinction between sensual and sexual when he publishes *Man and Woman* in 1966. Finally, he offers the distinction in German when he publishes *Die Enzyklika "Humanae Vitae"* in 1968. In this latter work, von Hildebrand often uses not *sinnlich* but the terms *sexuell* and *geschlechtlich*, both of which translate as "sexual." While von Hildebrand offers no explanation for the terminological shift, he seems to use *sinnlich* in his earlier writings to emphasize that a virtuous man is not one who remains unmoved by sensual desire but one whose desires are properly ordered to the created hierarchy of values (*Purity*, 27-39). Then, in his later writings, he distinguishes between *sinnlich* and *sexuell* and uses the latter

term when speaking specifically of man's sexual sphere. Although the translator of *Purity* does well to distinguish between *sinnlich* as meaning sexual and *sinnlich* as meaning sensual, I contend that he errs in dropping "sphere" from his translation of *die sinnliche Sphäre*. Accordingly, when the translator renders *die sinnliche Sphäre* as "sex" or "physical sex," I place "the sexual sphere" in brackets to indicate that von Hildebrand is referring to a sphere and not an action.

2. Von Hildebrand even indicates that consummation is implied by marriage when he writes: "Who can fail to grasp the grandeur and beauty of marriage *and the bodily union which it essentially implies* if he contemplates without prejudice the words of the Lord referring to the indissolubility of marriage?" (*The Encyclical "Humanae Vitae,"* 23, italics my own).

3. *Man and Woman*, 81; see also *The Encyclical "Humanae Vitae,"* 7. Consummation further fulfills the intention for union characteristic of conjugal love and promised in marital consent (*Man and Woman*, 81). For more discussion of the role consent and consummation play in conferring the sacrament of marriage, see Peter Elliott, *What God Has Joined . . . The Sacramentality of Marriage* (Staten Island, New York: Alba House, 1990), 84-87.

4. The 1917 Code of Canon Law, the *ius vigens* ("law in force") while von Hildebrand wrote on marriage issues, states: "A ratified and consummated valid marriage can be dissolved by no human power and for no cause, outside of death. . . . a non-consummated marriage between the baptized or [a marriage] between a baptized party and a non-baptized party can be dissolved by law upon solemn religious profession, or by dispensation granted by the Apostolic See for a just cause if both parties or [just] one ask for it, even if the other is unwilling" (*The 1917 Pio-Benedictine Code of Canon Law*, trans. Edward N. Peters [San Francisco, CA: Ignatius Press, 2001], canons 1118-1119, brackets in work cited). The ability of the Apostolic See to dissolve non-consummated marriages is known as the Petrine privilege. Note that the phrase concerning religious profession is not present in canon 1142 of the 1983 code where the Petrine privilege is mentioned. One should also note that while the dissolution of a non-consummated marriage is possible: "They invalidly attempt marriage who are bound by a prior bond, even if it is not consummated, with due regard for the privilege of the faith" (*Pio-Benedictine Code*, canon 1069, §1; see also canon 1085, §1 of the 1983 Code, *Code of Canon Law, Latin-English Translation: New English Translation*, trans. Canon Law Society of America [Washington, D.C.: Canon Law Society of America, 1999]).

5. *Marriage*, 20; see also *The Encyclical "Humanae Vitae,"* 7.

6. See the discussion of the Pauline privilege in chapter one.

7. *Pio-Benedictine Code*, canon 1119; see also canons 1142 and 1697-1698 of the 1983 Code.

8. All Scripture quotations come from the New American Bible.

9. *Man and Woman*, 88-89; see also 87, *The Encyclical "Humanae Vitae,"* 9, and *Purity*, 18, 40-41.

10. *Purity*, 41, italics in work cited, brackets my own.

11. *Purity*, 41.

12. Von Hildebrand repeatedly affirms that the conjugal act ought to be reserved for marriage; see *Purity*, 15-16; *Man and Woman*, 87; and *The Encyclical "Humanae Vitae,"* 7.

13. *Man and Woman*, 29.

14. *Purity*, 22.

15. *Purity*, 10, brackets my own; see also11-12, 13 and 18, and *Man and Woman*, 8.

16. *Purity*, 9; see also *Man and Woman*, 8 and *Marriage*, 15-16.

17. *Purity*, 12; see also *Purity*, 13 and 18; "Lambeth-Botschaft," 27; and *The Encyclical "Humanae Vitae,"* 23.

18. *Purity*, 5; see also 7 and *Man and Woman*, 18 and 88.

19. *Marriage*, 20, italics in work cited.

20. *Purity*, 5; see also 7; *Man and Woman*, 21; and Dietrich von Hildebrand and William A. Marra, *Sex Education: The Basic Issues* (St. Paul, MN: The Wanderer Press, 1969), 10.

21. *Purity*, 5; see also 7 and 22; *Man and Woman*, 21; and *Sex Education*, 10.

22. *Man and Woman*, 25. Von Hildebrand does not refer to any specific Scripture passage.

23. *Purity*, 3.

24. *Purity*, footnote, 6.

25. *Purity*, footnote, 6.
26. *Purity*, footnote, 6.
27. *The Encyclical "Humanae Vitae,"* 22. Note the similarity of von Hildebrand's remarks with Karol Wojtyla's analysis of shame as presented in *Love and Responsibility*, trans. H. T. Willetts (San Francisco, CA: Ignatius Press, 1993), 174-93; see especially 174, where Wojtyla writes, "We must not oversimplify the matter by maintaining that people endeavor to conceal only what is regarded as bad—for we often feel 'ashamed' of what is good." See also 179, where Wojtyla writes, "The function of shame is to exclude—(whether passively, as is usual with women, or actively, as is more often the case with men)—an attitude to the person incompatible with its essential, supra-utilitarian nature. The danger of such an attitude arises precisely because of the sexual values inherent in the person, and so sexual shame takes the form of a tendency to conceal them. This is a natural and spontaneous tendency. We see clearly here how the moral order is bound up with the existential order, the order of nature." While Wojtyla does not quote or reference von Hildebrand, their similarities here and elsewhere indicate that von Hildebrand's works may have exerted influence on the thought of Wojtyla. Since Wojtyla wrote considerably later than von Hildebrand, Wojtyla may have read von Hildebrand or he may have been influenced by von Hildebrand through the Catholic tradition. Another possible link is the influence that Max Scheler's writings had on both thinkers. Wojtyla mentions the influence of Scheler in his chapter on the "Metaphysics of Shame" (*Love and Responsibility*, 174) and von Hildebrand's close relationship with Scheler is well documented in von Hildebrand's biography: Alice von Hildebrand, *The Soul of a Lion* (San Francisco, CA: Ignatius Press, 2000), 69-111 and 146-49.
28. Von Hildebrand's conviction that the sexual sphere is a private secret to be protected has implications in his analysis of public "sex education." He writes, "Because the so-called sex education in the classroom deals with sex as a neutral topic of information such as spelling, it distorts the true nature of sex, not only because of its falsified content, but also because of the publicity which is fatal to the real, reverent grasping of the nature of sex. The scientist superstition here joins forces with the loss of all *discretio*, that is, the sense for the intimacy and privacy which certain topics require, and together they produce this abomination called sex education" (*Sex Education*, 18, italics in work cited).
29. *Purity*, 27.
30. *Purity*, 30.
31. *Purity*, 31, italics in work cited.
32. *Purity*, 25, brackets my own. Although the anonymous translator of *Purity* generally does well to distinguish when von Hildebrand's use of *sinnlich* is best translated as "sexual" and when it is best translated as "sensual," I place sensual in the third bracket of this quotation because here von Hildebrand appears to use *sinnlich* to mean sensuality in general and not sexuality in particular.
33. For more discussion of von Hildebrand's distinction between the virtue of purity and the temperament of insensuousness, see *Purity*, 31-37.
34. *Purity*, 27 and 30.
35. See *Purity*, 12 and 62, where von Hildebrand emphasizes that spouses must consciously focus on actualizing conjugal love in order to direct appropriately their sexual desire. Sexual desire is not bestial. The loss of one's freedom to sexual desire, that is, being dragged around by one's desire is what mimics the animals. Note the difference between von Hildebrand and Augustine on this point. Whereas von Hildebrand maintains that sexual desire can be properly directed by conjugal love, Augustine maintains that sexual desire is always evil. Only when the spouses aim to have children may the conjugal act be justified. Augustine writes, "intercourse of marriage for the sake of begetting *hath not fault*; but for the satisfying of lust, but yet with husband or wife, by reason of the faith of the bed, it hath venial fault: but adultery or fornication hath deadly fault" (*The Good of Marriage*, 402, italics my own).
36. *Purity*, 17; see also *Man and Woman*, 90-91, where von Hildebrand writes that, "we should read the *Canticle of Canticles*, open-mindedly . . . in its original literal sense; then we can breathe the atmosphere of this love, and see the sublimity of the bodily union when experienced as the ultimate God-given mutual self-donation."
37. *Purity*, 7; see also *Marriage*, 20, *Man and Woman*, 18, 87, and 88.

38. *Man and Woman*, 87; see also 18.
39. *Marriage*, 26; see also 21.
40. *Marriage*, 20, 21, 25-26, *Purity*, 13, and *Man and Woman*, 81.
41. *Man and Woman*, 47.
42. *Marriage*, 24.
43. *Purity*, 5, 16, and 31-39.
44. *Purity*, 11-12 and *Man and Woman*, 20.
45. *Purity*, 21.
46. *Purity*, 32.
47. *Man and Woman*, 92.
48. *Purity*, 38-39.
49. *Purity*, 47.
50. *Marriage*, 13.
51. *Purity*, 23.
52. *Marriage*, 13.
53. *Purity*, 33.
54. *Purity*, 23 and 43.
55. *Purity*, 17; see also 26.
56. *The Encyclical "Humanae Vitae,"* 9; see also 7, *Purity*, 15 and 16, and *Man and Woman*, 29 and 88-89.
57. *Purity*, 17, italics in work cited.
58. Von Hildebrand summarizes these three dispositions as well as the proper disposition of love in *Purity*, 28-29.
59. See *Ethics*, 295-311. For a brief distinction between the material and the vital-corporeal as applied to sexual union, see his footnote in *Purity*, 61.
60. *Purity*, 62.
61. To illustrate the danger of one's spirit being overwhelmed by his vital-corporeality, one can imagine that two friends go for a run—one is a runner and the other is not. As the run continues the runner begins talking to his friend about something important. The friend, however, struggles to pay attention because he is becoming short of breath. Finally, the exertion of the run demands his full attention so that he no longer hears what the runner is saying. In such a case the friend does not have complete moral responsibility for his inability to listen to the runner. Nonetheless, he did not enter fruitfully into the discussion and once the runner discovers his friend was not listening, he immediately recognizes the discussion was stripped of its most significant meaning, namely mutual exchange. The runner and the friend need to make sure that both parties are prepared to run and talk if they want to have a meaningful conversation.
62. *Purity*, 62. Augustine also provides a warning about the danger of sex: "So intense is the pleasure that when it reaches its climax there is an almost extinction of mental alertness; the intellectual sentries, as it were, are overwhelmed" (*City of God*, trans. Henry Bettenson [London: Penguin Books, 1984], 577). However, for Augustine, sexual desire is so disordered that it cannot be properly ordered: "The genital organs have become as it were the private property of lust, which has brought them so completely under its sway that they have no power of movement if this passion fails, if it has not arisen spontaneously or in response to a stimulus" (p. 581; see also 586). Whereas von Hildebrand maintains that the human spirit can direct the sexual drive, Augustine maintains that lust is present in every expression of the conjugal act even when the action leads to procreation (*City of God*, 580; see also *On the Good of Marriage*, 399, 404, and 412).
63. *Purity*, 25, italics in work cited; von Hildebrand proposes that this consciousness is required even if spouses intend to have children through their expression of the conjugal act: "the mere will to procreation is incapable of introducing into the act of wedded union the requisite element of conscious experience" (*Purity*, 13-14). Von Hildebrand further asserts that "even if the intention to reproduce were invested with the noble purpose of giving the Church new souls, that intention by itself, to the exclusion of specific wedded love, could not organically unite physical sex with the heart and spirit, nor would it possess the power to inform from within the distinctive nature of sex, alloyed as it is by a tendency to overcome the spirit"

(*Purity*, 14). One should note, however, that in *Marriage* von Hildebrand asserts that the "general connection between procreation and the communion of love must always be maintained even subjectively, at least as a general possibility of this act" (p. 23). This indicates that consciousness of procreation should play a role in expression of the conjugal act even if one's intention in expressing the conjugal act should not be reduced to procreation.

64. *Man and Woman*, 26; for more on von Hildebrand's discussion of the need for consciousness in moral action, see von Hildebrand, *Transformation in Christ*, trans. anonymous (San Francisco, CA: Ignatius Press, 1990), 53-69 and *Ethics* (New York: David McKay, 1953), 257-81.

65. *Purity*, 41. Von Hildebrand repeatedly speaks of the lover's surrender to the beloved (*Purity*, 5, 7, 21, 22; *Marriage*, 20; *Man and Woman*, 21; *Sex Education*, 10; *The Encyclical "Humanae Vitae,"* 7).

66. For a fuller discussion of the distinction between a giving into desire and a genuine self giving, with emphasis on the need to give one's self to God, see von Hildebrand's chapter on "True Surrender of Self" in *Transformation in Christ*, 481-500.

67. *Purity*, 28.

68. *Purity*, 29.

69. *Man and Woman*, 24.

70. *Man and Woman*, 30-31.

71. He writes, "there is no point in discussing the immorality of lechery with someone who is blind to the very nature and meaning of sex" (*Man and Woman*, 7).

72. *Man and Woman*, 8.

73. *Purity*, 21. Note also that in his work on *Man and Woman*, von Hildebrand identifies a further misuse of sex. Like diabolic lust this misuse involves not merely the disregarding of one of the conjugal act's characteristics but an isolation of one feature, namely mutuality, to the neglect of all others (*Man and Woman*, 26-27).

74. After discussing the misuse of the sexual sphere that occurs when one gives into sexual desire, von Hildebrand writes, "Even greater is the contrast between sex as the mystery of love and sex as the vehicle of diabolically evil lust" (*Purity*, 18); see also *Purity*, 23, 24; *Man and Woman*, 87. Von Hildebrand's distinction between the mere pursuit of sexual pleasure and the value of wedded love has a foundation in his graduate thesis and dissertation (this dissertation later was published as "Die Idee der sittlichen Handlung,"*Jahrbuch für Philosophie und phänomenologische Förschung*, 3 (1916): 126-251. Von Hildebrand made a contribution to values ethics by distinguishing between the manner in which an intrinsic value and something merely subjectively satisfying motivates a moral agent to action (*The Soul of a Lion*, 116-17). This distinction maintains a central place in von Hildebrand's writings. He gives the topic full discussion in his, *Ethics*, 34-63; see also his treatment of the legitimate pursuit of the subjectively satisfying, *Ethics*, 427-30. Von Hildebrand affirms that sexual desire is good, but he argues that affirming the goodness of the desire does not legitimize the reduction of the sexual sphere to instinct to the neglect of conjugal love (*Man and Woman*, 91). Pleasure should not be pursued to the neglect of intrinsic values.

75. For von Hildebrand, the denial of morality has severe consequences. He writes, "the amoral man has condemned himself to the periphery and finds no way back when he commits something objectively immoral. . . . the one who approaches the world having extinguished the light of morality, moves in a dull, falsified world, without depth, without thrill, without grandeur" (*Man and Woman*, 30-31).

76. *Purity*, 21 and 22; concerning the degradation of the other person involved in sexual union, see also *Man and Woman*, 27.

77. *Purity*, 22, italics in work cited.

78. *Purity*, 22. Other examples of desecration that von Hildebrand lists on the same page include violence to the human person's dignity, the money changers in the temple, and receiving Holy Communion for worldly motives.

79. *Purity*, 22; see also *Man and Woman*, 27.

80. *Purity*, 22.

81. *Purity*, 22.

82. *Purity*, 24.

83. *Purity*, 22; see also 23 and 45.
84. *Purity*, 23.
85. *Man and Woman*, 23.
86. *Man and Woman*, 22-23.
87. *Purity*, 69.
88. *Purity*, 68.
89. *Purity*, 71.
90. *Purity*, 70; see also 67-69.
91. *Purity*, 71.
92. *Purity*, 71.
93. *Purity*, 71.
94. *Purity*, 71.
95. *Purity*, 71-72.
96. *Purity*, 17.
97. *Purity*, 72-73 and 70-71; see also *Man and Woman*, 90 and *The Encyclical "Humanae Vitae,"* 10 and 11. Augustine acknowledges that lust can be tempered but he affirms this in relation to parental affections and not conjugal affections (*The Good of Marriage*, 400). Moreover, Augustine's idea of tempering lust involves the decrease of sexual desire rather than a proper ordering of that desire.
98. See *Man and Woman*, 25, where von Hildebrand writes, "The depth and existential impact of the bodily union also discloses itself if one realizes that to this deepest expression of love is confided the coming into existence of a new human being." See also *Purity*, 40-41 and "Lambeth-Botschaft," 26-28.
99. *Purity*, 15.

Chapter Three

The Primary Meaning of Marriage

Von Hildebrand, in his works on *Purity* and *Marriage*, sought to put conjugal love in its proper place. He did not, however, want to neglect the role of procreation in the process. Accordingly, he proposed that conjugal love is the primary meaning of marriage even while procreation is the primary end.[1] In line with the 1917 Code of Canon Law, many canon lawyers and theologians in the early twentieth century were accustomed to thinking of marriage in terms of the hierarchy of ends, with procreation being primary and mutual help and *remedia concupiscentia* being secondary.[2] Von Hildebrand's proposal that conjugal love is the primary meaning of marriage raises a number of questions concerning both the canonical hierarchy of ends and marriage in general.

In this chapter, my principal goal is not to answer these questions but to show how von Hildebrand's writings raise these questions in a new way. In doing so, I summarize commentary on von Hildebrand's distinction between primary meaning and primary end and offer my own commentary. Then, drawing on the analysis of conjugal love above, I attempt to explain what von Hildebrand means by asserting that conjugal love is the primary meaning of marriage.

A. FAILURE TO CLARIFY THE MEANING OF MEANING

A number of those who review von Hildebrand's English publication of *Marriage* express uncertainty about what he means in proposing that conjugal love is the primary meaning of marriage. Robert Hewitt wrestles with the concept on paper and warns against the lack of clarity he finds: "Is it strictly true to say that marriage *is* conjugal love, in the sense that it is its primary meaning? Does the author intend by the phrase 'primary meaning' what the Holy Father terms 'basis'?"[3] Since von Hildebrand writes *Marriage* for "the general public," Hewitt proposes that von Hildebrand's failure to clarify terms is particularly problematic.[4] Hewitt concludes, "We fear the general public will find the insistence upon the phrase 'primary meaning' a bit confusing."[5]

Another reviewer indicates that the concept "meaning" is not the only term he struggles to understand. He writes that *Marriage* "is not easy reading" and continues by saying, "Some may even suspect the work of belonging to a certain class of German writing of the last generation, which reveled in a metaphysical verbiage that, not infrequently, served as a smokescreen for concealing paucity and unclarity of ideas."[6] In the end, this reviewer seems to blame the translation for the lack of clarity. He writes of "an apparent reluctance on the part of the English translation to depart from the grammatical pattern of the original" and further states, "Dr. von Hildebrand, of course, needs no defense against any such charge. He belongs in the front rank of our best Catholic thinkers today."[7]

One reviewer (whose name is listed as M.P.B.) suggests that von Hildebrand's lack of clarity on the concept of meaning is a type of "fence-straddling."[8] The reviewer proposes that von Hildebrand "touches a current theological discussion" and that von Hildebrand "deliberately lays aside any discussion of it."[9] The same reviewer writes, "In this country von Hildebrand is well known for his *previous* works, *In Defense of Purity* and *Liturgy and Personality*" and proposes that von Hildebrand's "whole discussion of marriage takes its inspiration from that noteworthy passage of Pope Pius XI in *De casto conubio*."[10] The reviewer apparently is not aware that the English translation of *Marriage* was published nearly a decade and a half after the original German publication and that the original was written prior to both *Liturgy and Personality* and *Casti connubii*. More importantly, he appears to think that von Hildebrand wrote *Marriage* after the debates surrounding Herbert Doms's work.

The sharpest criticism comes from the pen of Bernard Lonergan. Lonergan summarizes von Hildebrand's proposal: "while the primary end of marriage is the procreation and education of children, the primary meaning of marriage is love."[11] Lonergan continues,

> The difficulty is the studied vagueness of the position. A book has been written on *The Meaning of Meaning*, and it concluded that 'meaning' has over eight hundred meanings. Which of these is meant by von Hildebrand, what is a primary meaning, what would be a secondary meaning, are so many questions conveniently left without an answer. So far is such lack of precision from Catholic philosophy and theology that it reminds one rather of Anglican comprehensiveness . . . it cannot be denied that he shares the romanticist vagueness and thinks in a misty middle distance where ideal love and plain fact merge.[12]

While one should not blame von Hildebrand for fence-straddling on debates that followed his work's publication, one can question why von Hildebrand refrains from defining a term central to his proposal.

B. WHAT IS THE MEANING OF MEANING?

Regardless of *why* von Hildebrand does not explain clearly his use of the phrase "primary meaning," he opens himself to misunderstanding by not defining his key terms. Therefore, one seeking to understand his use of "primary meaning" does well to explain his positive affirmations in relation to what he does *not* mean by the phrase, namely, that conjugal love is arbitrarily related to marriage, a synonym for marriage, or the primary end of marriage.

When von Hildebrand first proposes that conjugal love is the primary meaning of marriage in *Die Ehe*, he writes, "Die Liebe ist der primäre Schöpfungssinn der Ehe (Love is the primary, created meaning of marriage)."[13] Unfortunately, *Schöpfung* is dropped in the English translation so that the proposal reads not as "the primary, *created* meaning of marriage" but as "the primary meaning of marriage."[14] The difference between *Schöpfungssinn* and *Sinn* is crucial. Von Hildebrand does not use meaning in a merely subjective sense of the term as if conjugal love is the primary meaning to von Hildebrand and not necessarily for anyone else. On the contrary, he roots the concept of meaning in God's intention for marriage. Marriage does not mean whatever one wants it to mean. Rather, God as Creator has endowed marriage with a particular meaning and man's task is to understand, respect, and live out that meaning.

Conjugal love, therefore, has an objective character in marriage in the sense that meaning refers to a constitutive aspect of marriage as determined by God. In this regard, one can see that conjugal love is necessary to marriage because God always demands this love from spouses. One who enters marriage without manifesting the seeds of conjugal love and respect for the spouse's value concludes marriage in a manner offensive to God. Similarly, one offends God who lives the married life in a manner that does not foster conjugal love with his spouse. This is true even in the case of a marriage of renunciation.[15] In such a marriage, however, the one who offends God is not the one who continues to serve his spouse but the one who does not live out his married commitment and therefore denies his wife the opportunity for conjugal love. Conjugal love, then, is essential to marriage in the sense that God always requires spouses to foster this type of love. The fostering of conjugal love is a moral necessity that is not cast aside by any arbitrary decision or desire of the spouses.

Some reviewers of *Marriage* propose that von Hildebrand affirms conjugal love to be essential in another way, that is, as that which is required for a marriage to exist. In other words, they claim that von Hildebrand equates conjugal love with marriage.[16] John Ford gives this position the most lengthy and articulate expression. Ford points to von Hildebrand's proposal that "Love is—as we saw before—the essence of the [marriage] relation."[17] Ford also notes, however, von Hildebrand's assertion that conjugal love is not necessary for marriage.[18] Ford maintains that von Hildebrand's position on the role of conjugal love is self-contradictory: "He says, first, that conjugal love is the essence of marriage, and then that it is frequently absent from marriage and often impossible to people who nevertheless are capable of marriage. If these statements can be reconciled, then the word essential must be given a new definition."[19]

Like Ford, Arjonillo argues that von Hildebrand does not explain clearly his proposal that conjugal love is the primary meaning of marriage.[20] Nonetheless, this critique does not prevent Arjonillo from pulling together von Hildebrand's implicit discussion of the concept meaning: "several affirmations reveal that by this word, the author is referring to some inherent intelligible value or an ontological constituent of an objective reality which characterizes or specifies the nature of such reality and permits it to be defined."[21] Arjonillo does not maintain that conjugal love *is* the definition of marriage but that a definition of marriage must include mention of conjugal love. The existence of marriage does not require conjugal love, but conjugal love is the authentic motivation for marriage and spouses are required to foster conjugal love for one another. Conjugal love is necessary for marriage morally even if not ontologically.

Grubb notes that Ford ironically proposes some twenty years later that essence does not imply that which is necessary for marriage to be.[22] In his joint work with Gerard Kelly on *Marriage Questions*, Ford speaks of procreation, rearing of children, mutual help, the remedy for concupiscence, and the fostering of conjugal love as "the essential ends of marriage."[23] When he describes his use of the phrase essential he explains that he "does not mean that the actual realization of any of them is essential to any given marriage. A marriage which produces no children is still a marriage."[24] He goes on to explain that even a marriage "where there is hatred instead of love . . . remains a true marriage in the sense that the essence of marriage is still there."[25] Since Ford identifies conjugal love as an essential end of marriage, he argues the same thing he critiques von Hildebrand for asserting, namely, that conjugal love is essential to marriage even though conjugal love need not be present in every marriage.[26]

Ford, however, contends that the ends are essential to marriage in the sense that "the marriage bond essentially consists in a right to the acts by which the ends are achieved."[27] Spouses have rights over one another, not in the sense that they are obligated to attain the ends of marriage but that they must perform actions ordered toward those ends. While Ford provides an answer to the very question he poses to von Hildebrand twenty years earlier, his explanation, nonetheless, of how conjugal love is essential to marriage differs from von Hildebrand's analysis. According to von Hildebrand, the moral requirement to cultivate conjugal love is not merely a juridical right rooted in a legal contract but a requirement rooted in the personal value of the beloved and the lover's personal relationship with God. Furthermore, unlike Ford, von Hildebrand describes conjugal love as a meaning of marriage and not as an end.

Arjonillo explains that the emphasis that many theologians and canon lawyers placed on the hierarchy of ends in marriage had a long-standing tradition in the Catholic Church. Augustine spoke of three goods of marriage and argued that procreation was the only acceptable motivation for entering marriage and for expressing the conjugal act. Further, Arjonillo writes:

> The Scholastic theologians, with the exception of Hugo St. Victor and St. Bonaventure, were unanimous in their opinion of the existence of a hierarchy among the ends of marriage, dividing them into primary and secondary ends and attributing the primacy to the procreation of children. Perhaps, it was St. Thomas who most strongly affirmed the primacy of the procreative end, asserting that the children as [sic] the most essential end of marriage.[28]

Arjonillo asserts, however, that a hierarchical presentation of marriage's ends did not receive official ecclesial sanction until the early twentieth century.

Arjonillo writes, "It should be reminded [sic] that the *Codex Iuris Canonicis* of 1917, was the first official ecclesiastical document which explicitly made use of the terms *primary* and *secondary*, and which synthesized all the traditional doctrine of the Church in its canon 1013 § 1."[29] Arjonillo contends that after the 1917 Code's publication many theologians maintained "that marriage is a mere society for having children, and whose essence is identified with the so called *ius in corpus*."[30] Von Hildebrand seems to share Arjonillo's observation. In the 1942 introduction to *Marriage*, he writes, "In stressing the primary *end* of marriage—procreation—certain theological treatises have overlooked the primary *meaning* of marriage, which is love."[31] Whether or not theologians after 1917 emphasized procreation to the neglect of the other goods of marriage or whether this emphasis was an innovation in the tradition is a topic worthy of further study. The relevance for analysis of von Hildebrand's account of procreation is to note the framework from which many reviewers approached his proposal.

A number of reviewers insist on placing conjugal love within marriage's hierarchy of ends and therefore conclude that only procreation and not conjugal love can be primary. They critique von Hildebrand's use of "primary meaning" by arguing that von Hildebrand does not offer "a clear-cut distinction between the end and the meaning of marriage."[32] Bruehl, for example, contends that the personal values which von Hildebrand highlights "can be, and have been, fitted into the old scheme which speaks of the primary and secondary ends of marriage."[33] He further argues that the distinction between meaning and end "seems to be of questionable validity because a society receives its meaning, nature or essence from the end."[34] Ford echoes this assessment when he argues, "Marriage is essentially a juridical bond consisting of rights and duties. One cannot tell what the essential meaning of that bond is until one knows the ends for which it was instituted."[35]

Despite their criticisms, however, both Bruehl and Ford recommend von Hildebrand's writings. Bruehl encourages readership of von Hildebrand's *Marriage* insofar as the book "appeals more strongly to the modern mind."[36] Similarly, Ford writes,

> In spite of these adverse criticisms, it is possible to be in sympathy with the general scope and intention of Dr. von Hildebrand's work. The book can be recommended to young married couples who are likely to profit by it. . . . The secondary ends, and the all-pervading property of conjugal love as a duty of the spouses, begin now to receive their proper emphasis. And Dr. von Hildebrand has been especially successful in the second part of his book in pointing out the supernatural implications of this love.[37]

Bruehl and Ford are ambivalent in their review. On one hand, they argue that von Hildebrand's affirmation about conjugal love as the primary meaning of marriage does not fit into the scheme of hierarchical ends in which procreation alone is primary. On the other hand, they affirm von Hildebrand's remarks on conjugal love and they note the broad appeal of his observations. In the end, they contend that no church teaching is at stake and they even recommend the book.

Von Hildebrand is familiar with Augustine's influential presentation of the three goods of marriage. He notes them in his work on *Purity*; however, he does so not to highlight the primacy of procreation but to argue that procreation is not the only good of marriage. He writes,

> It is quite impossible to regard the union of love and sex in marriage as due exclusively to its aim of propagation. We should not forget that the Church assigns three ends to marriage, which St. Augustine sums up by the words *proles, fides, sacramentum*—offspring, fidelity, the sacrament. There exists, however, a profound relation of quality between the bodily union and that psychological and spiritual factor of specifically matrimonial love formulated under the terms *mutuum adjutorium* (mutual assistance), and *fides* (fidelity) as one of these three ends.[38]

Here, von Hildebrand identifies conjugal love with *fides* and therefore appears to place conjugal love within the hierarchy of ends. However, his emphasis is that procreation is not the *only* good of marriage, not to argue that conjugal love is one of the *ends* subordinate to procreation, a point highlighted by the fact that von Hildebrand repeatedly affirms that the fundamental relation of conjugal love to marriage is one of meaning and not end.

Von Hildebrand's distinction between meaning and end is not a clever attempt to subvert the hierarchy of ends in marriage. Rather, as Arjonillo asserts,

> Love was not identified with mutual help, nor was there a subtle desire to justify a separation between the unitive and procreative aspects of the conjugal act, which he categorically affirmed as a grave sin. On the contrary, von Hildebrand intended to insist on the proper manner by which marriage and procreation be [sic] understood. The distinction between meaning and end (and the difference between instrumental finality and finality of superabundance) were necessary in order to avoid identifying marriage as a mere means for procreation.[39]

Albert Schmitt notes in his review of *Die Ehe* that von Hildebrand distinguishes between meaning and end to highlight the centrality of conjugal love in marriage without downplaying the primacy of procreation. Schmitt writes, "one finds in many books of this kind, changes and expressions which are, only with difficulty, compatible with Church teaching. Von Hildebrand knows to avoid incompatibility with Church teaching by distinguishing between the meaning and end of marriage."[40]

I contend with Arjonillo that von Hildebrand's use of the term "meaning" is that which is constitutive of a thing, or that which is necessary to render a thing intelligible. Arjonillo relates von Hildebrand's remarks to Karol Wojtyla's use of the term in *Love and Responsibility* and the Fathers of the Second Vatican Council use of the term in *Gaudium et spes*. Wojtyla identifies love with the personalistic norm.[41] He explains the relationship between the personalistic norm (and therefore love) and ends as follows: "The personalistic norm itself is not, of course, to be identified with any one of the aims of marriage: a norm is never an end, nor is an end a norm. It is, however, a principle on which the proper realization of each of the aims mentioned, and of all of them together, depends."[42]

Similarly, Arjonillo explains that the Fathers of the Second Vatican Council refer to conjugal love not as an end of marriage but as the form,[43] life-giving principle,[44] unitive principle,[45] and vitality of marriage.[46] Arjonillo writes,

> According to von Hildebrand's thought, conjugal love serves as principal motor of marriage. . . . It is the élan, the vital impulse of marriage which is ordained toward the natural and supernatural perfection of the spouses. Love is seen as a vital principle of marriage: although conjugal love does not establish the marital bond, its existence makes marriage and conjugal life desirable. Without love, however, marriage would not fulfill the plans wanted by God. On the other hand, marriage protects the life of conjugal love.[47]

Arjonillo concludes that von Hildebrand's remarks "on conjugal love as a unifying and life-giving principle in marriage is consistent with the doctrine of the Council."[48]

Arjonillo's argument that the Fathers of the Second Vatican Council and von Hildebrand identify love not as an end but as the motivation and vitality of marriage is a key point in relation to statements made by Pope Pius XII. Pius XII repeatedly affirms that procreation is the primary end and that the other goods of marriage are subordinate to procreation. In a Decree of the Holy Office in 1944, Pius XII states,

> The Most Excellent and Reverend Fathers of this Supreme congregation, charged with the defense of the faith and morals, met on Wednesday, March 29, 1944, to consider the following question: 'Whether the opinion of some current authors is admissible which either denies that the primary end of marriage is the generation and nurture of offspring, or teaches that the secondary ends are not essentially subordinate to the primary, but are independent of it and equally primary.' Our response to this in decree: negative.[49]

If von Hildebrand had proposed that conjugal love was an end greater or equal to procreation, his remarks would have stood in tension with this strong affirmation of Pius XII. However, since von Hildebrand treats conjugal love not as an end but as the motivation and vitality of marriage, he is free from Pius's rebuke.

Von Hildebrand, in his early work, *Marriage*, proposes that conjugal love is the primary meaning of marriage. He perhaps meant by the phrase that conjugal love is constitutive of marriage as the authentic motivation for marriage and the vitality of marriage, that conjugal love is the constitutive moral norm of marriage upon which the other aims of marriage depend. Nonetheless, von Hildebrand's main focus is not to show that conjugal love is the "primary meaning" of marriage. He asserts the claim and does not develop an argument showing how something can have primary meaning. Further, he drops use of the phrase "primary meaning" in his later works, *Man and Woman* and *The Encyclical "Humanae Vitae."* His focus rather was to show that conjugal love should not be reduced to procreation and to describe the role of conjugal love in marriage.

C. SUMMARY

As many of the early reviewers indicate, von Hildebrand does not explain clearly his proposal that conjugal love is the "primary meaning" of marriage. This lack of clarity opens von Hildebrand's writings to possible misunderstandings. One is left then to bring together various statements that von

Hildebrand offers to clarify what he does and does not mean by the phrase. First, von Hildebrand does not intend by the term "meaning" something merely subjective in the sense that marriage is whatever one wants it to be. Rather, von Hildebrand argues that marriage's meaning has an objective character determined by the meaning given to it by God.

Second, von Hildebrand does not equate conjugal love with marriage. Conjugal love is the essence of marriage not as that which must be present for marriage to exist, but as that which is constitutive of marriage. Although von Hildebrand identifies conjugal love with one of the ends of marriage, he does so in passing to indicate that procreation is not the only good of marriage. He insists that the fundamental relation between conjugal love and marriage is a relationship of meaning.

By bringing von Hildebrand's remarks together one can see that conjugal love carries a primary character as motivation, as morally required in marriage, as the vitality of marriage, and as necessary to render marriages intelligible. Overall, von Hildebrand appears less concerned with showing how conjugal love is primary and more concerned with showing the significance of conjugal love in a way that does not undermine procreation's role in marriage. In fact, von Hildebrand discontinues use of the phrase "primary meaning" after the English translation of his work on *Marriage*. In his later works, von Hildebrand simply discusses conjugal love as relating to the meaning of marriage and he highlights conjugal love as the motivation and foundation of marriage.

To be sure, von Hildebrand does not deny that conjugal love is the primary meaning of marriage in these later writings. On the contrary, he continues to stress the centrality of conjugal love. By dropping the phrase "primary meaning" in his later writings, von Hildebrand avoids giving the impression that procreation no longer has a primary role in marriage. Nonetheless, von Hildebrand maintains that one should not downplay conjugal love simply because of possible misunderstandings. On the contrary, he insists that an adequate treatment of conjugal love enhances rather than diminishes the role of procreation in marriage.

Notes

1. *Marriage*, v, vi, 4, and 21. Von Hildebrand somewhat anticipates this proposal in *Purity*, when he writes that in addition to the end of marriage, the conjugal act also has the meaning of conjugal love (*Purity*, 12; see also *Reinheit*, 25). The original German words for the terms "meaning" and "end" are respectively *Sinn* and *Zweck*. While the English translation of *Purity* uses the terms "significance" and "object" instead of "meaning" and "end" I have elected to use meaning and end because this seems closer to von Hildebrand's use and because this is how the terms are translated in *Marriage*. One can find another early formulation of von Hildebrand's distinction between meaning and end in his response article to the 1930 Lambeth Conference. Von Hildebrand writes, "The essential meaning of marriage is the mutual love, the 'becoming one' in love, and the reciprocal raising to eternal destiny; the essential end is the generation of a new man" (Lambeth-Botschaft, 21, my translation; the original reads as follows: "Ist die

gegenseitige Liebe, das 'Einswerden' in Liebe und das gegenseitige Sich-emportragen zur ewigen Bestimmung der eigentliche Sinn der Ehe, so ist die Erzeugung neuer Menschen der eigentliche Zweck derselben"). Arjonillo suggests that von Hildebrand draws the general distinction between meaning and end from Max Scheler, but indicates that von Hildebrand is the first to apply the distinction to marriage (Arjonillo, 46).

2. Canon 1013, §1 of the 1917 Code of Canon Law: "The primary end of marriage is the procreation and education of children; the secondary [end] is mutual support and a remedy for concupiscence" (*The 1917 Pio-Benedictine Code of Canon Law*, trans. Edward N. Peters [San Francisco, CA: Ignatius Press, 2001], brackets in work cited). The 1983 code does not retain the language of primary and secondary ends (*Code of Canon Law, Latin-English Translation: New English Translation*, trans. Canon Law Society of America [Washington, D.C.: Canon Law Society of America, 1999], canons 1055-1056).

3. Robert A. Hewitt, review of *Marriage*, by Dietrich von Hildebrand, *America* 67 (6 June 1942): 244, italics in work cited.

4. Hewitt, 244. Hewitt's remark is based on the preface von Hildebrand wrote to the English publication of his own work, *Marriage*: "Unlike *In Defense of Purity* by the same author, this work is exclusively concerned with marriage and is addressed to a general public" (p. vii, note that while von Hildebrand is referred to in the third person, he is the author of this preface).

5. Hewitt, 244.

6. G.L.D., review of *Marriage*, by Dietrich von Hildebrand, *Oratre Fratres* 16 (14 June 1941): 382. The full name of the reviewer is not listed.

7. G.L.D., 382. One should note that other reviewers disagree with G.L.D. both on the issue of technical language and the quality of the translation. A reviewer identified as M.P.B. writes, "Its untechnical language and treatment makes it a 'must' book for every educated Catholic who endeavors to keep well read" (M.P.B., review of *Marriage*, by Dietrich von Hildebrand. *Dominicana* 27 [October 1942]: 190). Concerning the translation, Kilian J. Hennrich writes, "The work here reviewed was originally written in German, but the translation is excellent" (Hennrich, review of *Marriage*, by Dietrich von Hildebrand, *Homiletic and Pastoral Review* 42 [1942]: 1078).

8. M.P.B., 190.

9. M.P.B., 189.

10. M.P.B., 189, italics my own; see also Grubb's discussion of this review, "Anthropology of Marriage," 130-31.

11. Bernard Lonergan, review of *Marriage*, by Dietrich von Hildebrand, in *Shorter Papers*, vol. 20 of *Collected Works of Bernard Lonergan*, ed. Frederick Crowe and Robert Doran (Toronto: University of Toronto Press, 2007), 155.

12. Lonergan, 155-56; see also Ford, review of *Marriage*, 545.

13. *Die Ehe*, 7, my translation.

14. *Marriage*, 4.

15. According to von Hildebrand, a marriage of renunciation is when one spouse seeks to foster conjugal love and the other does not. The lover must remain faithful to his spouse even if this means renouncing the possibility of authentic conjugal love; see von Hildebrand's *Marriage*, 30-32 and 47.

16. See John C. Ford, review of *Marriage*, by Dietrich von Hildebrand, *Thought* 17 (September 1942): 544-45; see also Hewitt, 244 and Grubb, 133-34, 280-81, and 301.

17. *Marriage*, 60, brackets are my own; Ford mentions this phrase on 544 of his review. Elsewhere, Ford writes that von Hildebrand, "makes conjugal love the primary meaning of marriage (presumably its essential meaning)" (John C. Ford, S.J. and Gerard Kelly, S.J., *Marriage Questions*, vol. 2 of *Contemporary Moral Theology* [Westminster, MD: Newman Press, 1964], 112).

18. Ford, review of *Marriage*, 544-45. See *Marriage*, 30-31, where von Hildebrand discusses marriages of renunciation, such as the marriage of Saint Monica, in which one spouse must remain faithful to her marriage commitment despite the other spouse who does not live out their marriage commitment and therefore undermines the mutuality necessary for conjugal love.

19. Ford, 544-45.
20. Arjonillo, 300.
21. Arjonillo, 300.
22. Grubb, 290-91. When Grubb notes that Ford commits the same error as von Hildebrand, Grubb is not justifying von Hildebrand but critiquing both thinkers. Grubb argues that conjugal love is essential to marriage in the sense that the validity of marriage requires the presence of conjugal love. In a somewhat surprising twist, Grubb writes in the concluding paragraph of his dissertation, "Von Hildebrand should have trusted his first instinct and its consequence: not everyone is capable of such a relationship and, as a result, not everyone is capable of sacramental marriage. Only where the true mutual donation and reception of persons is possible (the anthropological factor), can the sacrament (the theological significance) be a possibility" (p. 301).
23. *Marriage Questions*, 49.
24. *Marriage Questions*, 49.
25. *Marriage Questions*, 49.
26. *Marriage Questions*, 117 and 121.
27. *Marriage Questions*, 57.
28. Arjonillo, 241, footnote 88.
29. Arjonillo, 242. Canon 1013 § 1 reads: "The primary end of marriage is the procreation and education of children; the secondary [end] is mutual support and a remedy for concupiscence" (*Pio-Benedictine Code*, brackets in work cited; the 1983 Code does not use the language of primary and secondary ends). See also canon 1081, § 2: "Matrimonial consent is an act of the will by which each party gives and accepts perpetual and exclusive rights to the body, for those actions that are of themselves suitable for the generation of children" (*Pio-Benedictine Code*; this code is not included in the 1983 *Code of Canon Law*) and canon 1082, § 1: "In order that matrimonial consent be considered [valid], it is necessary that the contractants at least not be ignorant that marriage is a permanent society between a man and woman for the procreation of children" (*Pio-Benedictine Code*, brackets in work cited; see also *Code of Canon Law,* canon 1096, § 1). Arjonillo mentions these latter two canons from the *Pio-Benedictine Code* in *Conjugal Love and the Ends of Marriage*, 38.
30. Arjonillo, 39, italics in work cited.
31. *Marriage*, vi, italics in work cited. Arjonillo contends that the emphasis on procreation to the neglect of marriage's other goods flows not from the Code but that "the doctrine found in this canon was radicalized by some canonists during the first half of the century up to the point of considering the secondary end of marriage as something accidental, i.e., not essential to marriage" (p. 39).
32. Edgar Schmiedeler, review of *Marriage*, by Dietrich von Hildebrand, *The Catholic Educational Review* 40 (October 1942): 509.
33. C. Bruehl, review of *Marriage*, by Dietrich von Hildebrand, *Commonweal* 36 (26 June 1942): 234. Unfortunately, Bruehl does not indicate how this might be done.
34. Bruehl, 234.
35. Ford, review of *Marriage*, 545. Similarly, Schmiedeler writes, "This reviewer fails to see a clear-cut distinction between the end and the meaning of marriage. A society receives its meaning, essence or nature from its end" (p. 509).
36. Bruehl, 234.
37. Ford, 545.
38. *Purity*, 7; see also 10-11 and John Noonan, *Contraception: A History of Its Treatment by Catholic Theologians and Canonists*, enlarged ed. (Cambridge, MA: Harvard University Press, 1986), 495.
39. Arjonillo, 343; see also Grubb, 280. Arjonillo explains that after von Hildebrand presented his distinction between meaning and end in a 1923 lecture, von Hildebrand "sought the consent of an ecclesiastical authority, His Eminence Cardinal Pacelli, the Papal Nuncio in Munich. Upon expounding his opinion to Cardinal Pacelli, von Hildebrand received the endorsement from the future Pope Pius XII" (Arjonillo, 53; see also *The Soul of a Lion*, 212). When Arjonillo writes that "love was not identified with mutual help" (p. 343), he either fails to acknowledge that von Hildebrand makes this identification or he is arguing that the identifi-

cation was not a true identification because von Hildebrand emphasizes the relationship between conjugal love and marriage as a relationship of meaning.

40. Albert Schmitt, review of *Die Ehe*, by Dietrich von Hildebrand, *Zeitschrift für katholische Theologie* 54 (1930): 309, my translation. The German reads as follows: "Freilich finden sich in manchen Büchern und Schriften dieser Art Wendungen und Ausdrücke, die mit der Lehre der Kirche nur schwer vereinbar sind. H. weiß das zu vermeiden durch die Unterscheidung von Zweck und Sinn der Ehe."

41. Wojtyla explains the personalistic norm as follows: "This norm, in its negative aspect, states that the person is the kind of good which does not admit of use and cannot be treated as an object of use and as such the means to an end. In its positive form the personalistic norm confirms this: the person is a good towards which the only proper and adequate attitude is love" (Karol Wojtyla, *Love and Responsibility*, trans. H. T. Willetts [San Francisco, CA: Ignatius Press, 1981], 41).

42. Wojtyla, 67; Wojtyla also writes, "With this in mind, it seems equally clearly indicated that the *mutuum adiutorium* mentioned in the teaching of the Church on the purposes of marriage as second in importance after procreation must not be interpreted—as it often is—to mean 'mutual love'. Those who do this mistakenly come to believe that procreation as the primary end is something distinct from 'love', as also is the tertiary end, *remedium concupiscentiae*, whereas both procreation and *remedium concupiscentiae* as purposes of marriage must result from love as a virtue, and so fit in with the personalistic norm. *Mutuum adiutorium* as a purpose of marriage is likewise only a result of love as a virtue" (*Love and Responsibility*, 67-68). Arjonillo points to Wojtyla's analysis in *Conjugal Love and the Ends of Marriage*, 236.

43. Arjonillo, 306.

44. Arjonillo, 298 and 308.

45. Arjonillo, 306.

46. Arjonillo, 308; Arjonillo also notes that according to Bernard Häring, "Conjugal love is 'not to be regarded as an end (*finis*) of marriage annexed to the other ends or set side by side with them. Married love is, by virtue of its inmost nature and form, the very force that serves new life'" (Arjonillo, 250, the inside quote is from Häring, *Community of love*, in Edna McDonagh, ed., *The Meaning of Christian Marriage* [Dublin: M. H. Gill and Son, 1963], 66-67).

47. Arjonillo, 308.

48. Arjonillo, 309.

49. Grubb, 170; quoted from S. S. Congregatio S. Officii, "Decretum de finibus matrimonii, 1 April 1944,"*AAS* 36 (1944): 103, the English translation of the decree is taken from Theodore Mackin, S.J., *What is Marriage?* (New York: Paulist Press, 1982), 235-36; see also Pope Pius XII, "The Apostolate of the Midwife," in *Major Addresses of Pope Pius XII*, vol. 1, ed. Vincent A. Yzermans (St. Paul, MN: North Central Publishing, 1961), 172; the translator is not listed; *AAS*, 43 (195): 848-49. Grubb notes that while Pius XII affirms that procreation is primary, he does not explain how procreation is primary and in what way the other goods of marriage are subordinate to procreation (Grubb, 171).

Part II

Procreation

Chapter Four

Reverence and Superabundance

In part two of his work *The Encyclical "Humanae Vitae,"* von Hildebrand deals with the topic of marriage and procreation. At the beginning of this section, he provides a perceptive summary of his account of procreation's role in marriage:

> To this sublime love union God has confided the coming into being of a new man, a cooperation with His divine creativity. Could we think of any thing more beautiful than this connection between the deepest love communion, the ultimate self-donation out of love, and the creation of a new human being? A deep mystery is here offered to us, which calls for reverence and awe. But we can grasp the grandeur and depth of this connection only if we first understand the meaning and value of marriage as a love communion and the meaning and value of the marital act as the consummation of this ultimate union to which spousal love aspires. We can appreciate the mysterious character of the link between the marital act and the birth of a new person only if we have understood its finality as an instance of the principle of superabundance and not as an instrumental finality in which the conjugal act is looked at as a mere means for procreation. And it must be most emphatically stated that understanding the meaning and value of marriage as a love union *does not minimize but rather enhances the link between marriage and procreation.*[1]

Von Hildebrand indicates that four things are necessary in order to understand the role of procreation is marriage. One must understand marriage as a love union, the role of the conjugal act as the consummation of marriage, reverence and awe, and the principle of superabundance. He then proposes that a proper understanding of marriage as a love union does not minimize but enhances the link between marriage and procreation. Since I have discussed conjugal love, marriage, and the conjugal act above, I now turn to von Hildebrand's discussion of superabundant finality, reverence, and then defend his proposal that his account of conjugal love enhances the link between marriage and procreation.

A. THE PRINCIPLE OF SUPERABUNDANCE

Although von Hildebrand's writings on marriage and sexual ethics have a remarkable consistency, one important development is his articulation of the principle of superabundance. In his later writings, *Man and Woman* and *The Encyclical "Humanae Vitae,"* he puts great stress on this principle proposing that one must understand procreation as a superabundant end in order to appreciate the mysterious link between marriage and procreation.[2]

Superabundance, understood in the general sense of the term, simply involves a going beyond, or an overflow of something. Conjugal love and love of God, for example, involve a temporal superabundance: "Conjugal love implies an intention of *going beyond* even the giving of self, which is inherent in love as such. It desires an objective self-giving once and for ever, an irrevocable giving which persists independently of all subjective inconstancy. . . . A similar superabundant love impels certain persons to give themselves once and for ever exclusively to God."[3] The present moment cannot contain these forms of love.

Von Hildebrand's discussion of *superabundant finality* involves a more specific "going beyond" than his general use of "superabundance." He explains superabundant finality in contrast to instrumental finality. The central distinction is the significance of the thing serving as a means: "In instrumental finality the being which is considered as means is in its meaning and value completely dependent upon the end, whereas in the superabundant finality, it has a meaning and value independently of the end to which it leads."[4] Elsewhere, von Hildebrand writes, "In instrumental finality, the end is the exclusive *raison d'être* of the means; in superabundant finality, the good serving the end has also a *raison d'être* in itself."[5] Superabundant finality is unique in that the means have significance beyond the ends they serve.

Von Hildebrand provides a number of examples to illustrate instrumental finality. Concerning a knife, he writes, "the end—cutting—determines its entire nature; its meaning is identical with serving this end, and its value depends upon its function as a means."[6] Other examples that he discusses are the use of a surgical instrument for operating, money for procuring a good, teeth for the mastication of food,[7] and an egg-shell in protecting a developing embryo.[8] In each case, the object is merely instrumental. Without reference to its end, it lacks meaning.

As an example of superabundant finality, von Hildebrand discusses participation in the liturgy. He proposes that one should enter into liturgy to give glory to God. The personal transformation that results from participation in liturgy is a superabundant fruit:

> The deepest *pedagogical* effect is achieved through that which is not used as a *pedagogical means*: It is achieved through that which, independent of pedagogical action, dispenses it as a *superfluum* or gift of superabundance. Thus the deepest and most organic transformation of man in the spirit of Christ is found precisely at that point where we purely respond to values, in the giving up of ourselves to God's glory, in the glorifying of God performed as divine service, in the abiding *Coram ipso* (in standing before him), in the rejoicing in God's existence, in the *Gloria Domini* (The glory of the Lord).[9]

One should not use God or the liturgy as a means to personal transformation; rather, one seeks to glorify God in the liturgy, and personal transformation superabundantly results.[10]

Central to superabundant finality is von Hildebrand's insight concerning the distinctiveness of value as something good in itself, a good never to be used merely as a means. One important implication of this insight is the personal moral consciousness required for all authentic value responses. In his work, *Transformation in Christ*, von Hildebrand explains true consciousness in relation to two forms of false consciousness.[11] In the first form of false consciousness, one destroys "the attitude of genuine absorption in the object by an excess of reflective self-observation."[12] If someone with this disposition "is listening to some beautiful music, he at once develops an awareness of his own reaction, and thus loses the possibility of a genuine response to that beautiful music."[13]

The second form of self-consciousness is a "tendency to over-intellectualism, implying that even in a situation which calls upon us to decide or to act rather than merely to know, we persevere in a purely cognitive attitude."[14] For example, "suppose a man sees someone in immediate danger of life, and, instead of rushing to his rescue, studies his facial expressions."[15]

True consciousness requires attentiveness to "the theme present in a given situation."[16] In liturgical celebration, the theme is the glorification of God. If one were caught up in self observation of personal growth to the neglect of God's glory, one would fall into the first form of false consciousness. Similarly, one commits a false intellectualism, who focuses on things, such as the color of the priest's vestments or who one will speak with after Mass, and thereby fails to enter into the liturgy.

The principle of superabundance involves a causal relationship but not an instrumental one. That is, the means that lead to the end are willed for their own sake and not merely as means to another end. The object that leads to an end, since it has value in itself, should be consciously sought for its own sake. In other words, not only do the means have value in themselves but the moral agent must be aware consciously of that value, an awareness that must manifest itself in the agent's action. The moral agent's consciousness should not be directed to the superabundant fruit in a manner that compromises the consciousness required toward the object that has value in itself.

Von Hildebrand proposes that the causal relationship between the conjugal act and procreation is superabundant: "The God-given, essential link between love of man and woman and its fulfillment in the marital union, on the one hand, and the creation of a new person, on the other hand, has precisely the character of superabundance, which is a much deeper connection than would be one of merely instrumental finality."[17] Human persons relate differently to procreation than do animals. Whereas for animals, the significance of physical sex is "functional in the narrowest sense," the relation between the conjugal act and procreation for man "cannot be purely utilitarian."[18]

While recognizing that biological laws connect the conjugal act with procreation, von Hildebrand argues that "The generation of a new human being, a spiritual person who is an image of God, clearly bears not only a biological value but also an eminently personal value."[19] The connection between the conjugal act and procreation has a *functional* relation in the sense that the conjugal act is biologically ordered toward procreation. However, this connection is not merely functional, that is, not *instrumentally functional* in the sense that the meaning of the conjugal act is reduced to procreation or that procreation is simply biological.

Human procreation, unlike the manner in which animals propagate, carries an important personal and inter-personal dimension. Von Hildebrand writes, "apart from the relation of physical sex to procreation (*procreatio*), there exists a relation arising out of their respective qualities between physical sex and wedded love, which constitutes the significance of the former for man *in quantum homo*."[20] Further, the conjugal act contains meaning unique to Christians as a participation "in the sacramental meaning of marriage."[21]

To clarify that procreation is not merely the instrumental result of the conjugal act, von Hildebrand even addresses the question from God's perspective. Some contend, he states, that even if spouses enter sexual union from the motivation of conjugal love "God has implanted in their hearts the love between man and woman and the desire for a conjugal union as a mere means for procreation."[22] In response, von Hildebrand distinguishes between experiences of urges or instincts and spiritual acts of the person. Concerning instincts, he gives the example of thirst: "its *raison d'être* is to procure for the body the necessary liquid . . . God has installed it as a means to that end."[23] Concerning spiritual acts of the person, he writes, "we can no longer assume that in the eyes of God they have no meaning in themselves. . . . The spiritual attitudes of man have a meaning and a *ratio* in themselves and they can never be treated as having their real significance independently of the person."[24]

Since conjugal love, marriage, and the conjugal act involve spiritual acts of the person, von Hildebrand argues that God does not use these actions as means to procreation: "Man is not a puppet for God, but a personal being to whom God addresses Himself and from whom He expects a meaningful response."[25] Marriage and conjugal love are not instruments to attain procreation; rather, procreation is a superabundant fruit.

Von Hildebrand's contention that marriage and the conjugal act have value in addition to procreation has a number of implications. He proposes, for example, that the community of marriage is in some ways superior to the family:

> The unifying principle here touches the deepest root of personal life. Here love is—as we saw before—the essence of the relation. Its principle embraces not only the most intimate happiness of each but also the mutual abandon of love, an ardent interest in the spiritual and moral growth of the beloved, an affirmation of the unique idea of God which is incarnated in the other person. This community involves man in his whole nature as does no other community. It extends to all spheres of life, from the most central to the peripheral.[26]

Marriage is superior to the family in the sense that marriage ought to be more essentially rooted in love, be more intimately related to man's happiness, and involve the spouses' whole being.

Accordingly, marriage remains meaningful and valid even when one or both spouses realize that they are infertile.[27] In his work on *Marriage*, von Hildebrand asks a series of rhetorical questions that presume the validity of marriages that are not blessed with the gift of a child: "Can a childless marriage be regarded as a failure, as something that did not fulfill its meaning? Can we justly assert that it would have been better if such a marriage had not been brought to pass? Can it not have its full divinely-appointed meaning simply as the highest communion of love, and glorifying God by this very fact?"[28] He answers these questions in part by arguing that a faithful and loving marriage without children fulfills the ideal of marriage to a higher degree than a marriage with children "where the partners are unfaithful to each other and desecrate the sacred tie by a lack of love and loyalty"[29]

Similarly, expressions of the conjugal act not resulting in procreation still retain value. Von Hildebrand writes, "The conjugal act does not in any way lose its full meaning and value if one knows that a conception is out of the question, as when age, or an inevitable operation for the sake of health, or pregnancy exclude it."[30] Even when procreation does not result, the conjugal act retains meaning as an actualization of conjugal love. If a conjugal act not leading to procreation "is an expression of a deep love, anchored in Christ, it will rank even higher in its quality and purity than one that leads to a conception in a marriage in which the love is less deep and not formed in Christ."[31] If procreation were the only meaning of the conjugal act, then "it would be incomprehensible, in the last analysis, why an illegitimate union should be sinful when children result from it."[32] Moral reflection on the conjugal act, in addition to its link with procreation, must consider the personal values of the spouses involved and the action's connection to marriage and to conjugal love.

Von Hildebrand highlights a few theological foundations for his position that marriage and the conjugal act have meaning when procreation does not result. He explains that the Genesis authors, when describing God's intention for creating woman, write in God's voice, "It is not good for man to be alone; let us make him a help like unto himself."[33] God's motivation for creating woman is man's loneliness and need for fellowship, not procreation.[34] Von Hildebrand further writes, "Is this not a clear indication that marriage is a symbol of the union of the soul with God, that it possesses, as such, a sublime importance and that it exists in the first place for its own sake and not exclusively for the sake of any result that it produces?"[35] For von Hildebrand, the theological affirmation that spouses image the union between God and the human soul comes into greater relief when one recognizes that the meaning of marriage is not reduced to procreation.

B. INTENTIONALITY IN SUPERABUNDANT FINALITY

Von Hildebrand's principle of superabundance is crucial for maintaining respect for values. Values require a due response and should never be used merely as a means to another good. Leaving the integrity of this insight in place, that a value should not be reduced to serving another good, one might wonder, where does that leave the goods that flow superabundantly from our actions? One should not reduce values to other goods but one must also avoid the error of proposing that an action's superabundant fruit must be denied or ignored in order to maintain the integrity of the relevant value.

This latter error comes into clarity when the superabundant fruit is intimately linked with the value under consideration. When entering into liturgy, one not only foresees that one will develop humility and piety but the development of these virtues cannot be separated from worshipping God. While one would do wrong to use worship merely as a means to grow in humility and piety, if liturgical worship is cultivating pride and impiety, then, one is failing to worship God. The growth of humility and piety does not happen by surprise, and more than being foreseen, such development is intimately related to and cannot be separated from liturgical worship.

Von Hildebrand's concept of superabundance raises questions about intentionality and the relationship between a value and the superabundant fruit it produces. One should note here that the difficulty of identifying an action's intention is by no means unique to von Hildebrand. Elizabeth Anscombe speaks to the issue's complexity in her work on *Intention*. She imagines a situation in which as she describes:

> A man is pumping water into the cistern which supplies the drinking water of a house. Someone has found a way of systematically contaminating the source with a deadly cumulative poison whose effects are unnoticeable until they can no longer be cured. The house is regularly inhabited by a small group of party chiefs, with their immediate families, who are in control of a great state; they are engaged in exterminating the Jews and perhaps plan a world war. The man who contaminated the source has calculated that if these people are destroyed some good men will get into power who will govern well, or even institute the Kingdom of Heaven on earth and secure a good life for all the people; and he has revealed the calculation, together with the fact about the poison, to the man who is pumping. The death of the inhabitants of the house will, of course, have all sorts of other effects; e.g., that a number of people unknown to these men will receive legacies, about which they know nothing.[36]

In such a situation, one might ask with Anscombe, what is the man's intention for acting? The man's arm is moving up and down, muscles are contracting and relaxing, certain substances are being generated by the nerve fibers, the moving arm is casting a shadowy image on a rockery that looks like a face peering out, and the clicking noises of the pump are making a noticeable rhythm.[37]

While all of these descriptions are true descriptions of what is taking place, Anscombe proposes that only "the question 'Why?' enables us to narrow down our descriptions of what the man is doing to a range covering all and only his intentional actions."[38] Why was the man pumping the water? To contract and relax arm muscles is not a sufficient answer to the question why. Perhaps, he wants to make money, to kill the lot inside, to enable better leaders to rise to power, to build up the Kingdom of Heaven.

By defining the intention of the action in terms of why the action is performed, Anscombe is not proposing that the intention is whatever the moral agent says it is; one can lie or even be mistaken about one's own true intention. While thinking one is calling a friend to grow in holiness, one might really be unloading repressed anger harbored from a completely unrelated incident. One cannot greet another with a brutal punch to the face and then claim one intended for the punch to be an affectionate greeting.

If one gives application to the question why an action is performed in the case of liturgical worship, one sees that the intention ought to be the glory of God. The glory of God should be one's motivation for entering into liturgy; God's glory should receive one's conscious attentiveness. Yet, if this be one's intention, then how should one stand in relation to growth in humility and piety?

Anscombe provides some guidance here as well. She distinguishes between intending something and willing something voluntarily. All intentions involve willing something voluntarily but not all willing voluntarily involves intention. Willing voluntarily is behavior done wantingly. Intention answers the question why the moral agent acts. One can will something voluntarily without intending it in a few ways. The moral agent might know a good will result but that good does not explain why the action was performed. This is the case when one goes to the grocery store to buy food, but voluntarily wills to see and speak with a friend who works at the store.

Another way to will a good voluntarily without intending the good would be to will the good without conscious awareness. This happens, for example, when a caregiver receives a phone call while playing with her toddler. An observant young child knows when his caregiver is not giving true consciousness to the task at hand and the caregiver gets frustrated when the toddler will not allow her the necessary attentiveness to enter into a phone conversation. The lack of conscious focus undermines both shared activities.

In liturgical worship, while one's intention should be God's glory, one also should voluntarily will to develop the virtues of humility and piety. One intends the value while simultaneously and voluntarily willing superabundant goods. In *The Nature of Love*, von Hildebrand clarifies how this simultaneity can happen in his discussion of super-actual stances.

A super-actual stance is a value commitment that remains even when one is not consciously focused on that value. Von Hildebrand discusses two types of super-actual stances distinguished by the role the stance plays in one's life.[39] In the first type, one's stance has enduring validity. Respect, for example, need not be at the forefront of our consciousness every moment in order to endure. The enduring character of one's respect for another manifests itself when one sees someone one has not thought about for some time and one's respect immediately comes into conscious focus.

The second type of super-actual stance, in addition to having enduring validity, involves a stance so significant and central to the person that the stance colors and modifies all situations. The modification of experience involved here is not the irrational influence of a repressed sub-conscious but the enlightening influence of a super-conscious commitment. The most profound example of this type of super-actual stance is love for God. When one grows in love for God, one sees all creation in a new light, not only because God is Creator and all things participate in God but also because of the fundamental commitment that love of God involves. Unlike the case with respect for another, this type of super-actual stance is such that one will desire conscious attentiveness to the relevant value after a time of focusing on some other value. While one need not consciously focus on God at every moment, one deceives one's self to think one loves God but never desires to consciously focus on Him.

In liturgy, one's consciously focused intention to glorify God does not prevent one's super-actual commitment to live a virtuous life. While one should consciously focus on glorifying God, one should still voluntarily will to develop the virtues of humility and piety. Further, these super-actual stances, more than being voluntarily willed, enlighten how God should be glorified so that, for example, one is less likely to worship God in a way that cultivates pride.

Since certain superabundant fruits are intimately linked with the relevant value, one cannot help but be aware that the superabundant fruit will result. To recognize that objective goods result from a value response does not entail a lack of attentiveness to the value or prevent an authentic value-response; rather, von Hildebrand argues that when objective goods are intimately related to a value response and we are aware of this connection, the value response becomes a super-value response. That the value brings us goodness and fulfillment manifests and actualizes our commitment to that value.[40]

Insofar as intention explains why someone is acting and the conscious focus of one's action, then one should not intend the superabundant fruit. This does not mean one must deny or ignore superabundant fruit. Rather, even more than foreseeing the fruit one should voluntarily will the superabundant fruit. Further, one's super-actual stances toward superabundant goods color how one responds to the relevant value.

The intention of the conjugal act should be one's beloved and the actualization of conjugal love. Conjugal love should be the motivation for the action and the conscious focus of the spouses during the action. At the same time, procreation is a good related essentially to the conjugal act. Spouses should not only foresee procreation, but they should voluntarily will this good in their expression of the conjugal act. Moreover, one's super-actual stance toward procreation should color how and when one expresses the conjugal act. On this latter point, one must be clear about what a super-actual stance toward procreation entails.

A super-actual stance toward procreation is less a commitment to someone who does not yet exist and more a commitment to God. Von Hildebrand explains in his defense of *Humanae vitae* that the expression of spousal love in the conjugal act relates to the virtue of purity whereas one's disposition toward procreation relates to the virtue of reverence.[41] To understand this claim, one needs to know what von Hildebrand means by the virtue of reverence. He does not mean merely saying one's first Friday devotion.

C. REVERENCE

Von Hildebrand provides an insightful discussion of the virtue of reverence in his works *Liturgy and Personality*[42] and *Art of Living*.[43] I will summarize his account and then analyze how he applies these insights to conjugal love, marriage, the conjugal act, and procreation.

Von Hildebrand proposes that the foundation of reverence is recognition of man's metaphysical situation, that is, man's fundamental status before God.[44] This metaphysical situation consists of three main characteristics. The first characteristic is "the fact that we have received 'all that we have and are'—except sin—from God."[45] God is Creator and man is created. The second characteristic is "the infinite distance between us and absolute Being."[46] God is all in all and man appears as nothing before Him. Third, whereas God is all-knowing and all-powerful, man has "debility and limitation."[47] In summary, one might say that the metaphysical situation is that man is man and God is God.

Fully developed reverence is based on one's right relationship with God.[48] Man must recognize that he is not God and that God is greater than himself. Accordingly, the reverent man does not seek to appropriate God and His creation for his own purposes and pleasures, but "is disposed to know something higher than himself and his pleasure, and wills to submit to it and abandon himself."[49] The temptation to falsely appropriate God for personal pleasure is not a temptation unique to vicious men but manifests itself even in those who aspire to glorify God: "How often, even in a religious man, do we find mixed in with his relations to God a certain self-relishing—so clearly shown wherever the relationship to God is a sentimental one."[50]

In order to stand in right relation to God, one must first grow in knowledge of God. One must recognize that to man God is a mystery. Man *does not* understand God fully and man *cannot* understand God fully. God is beyond man's capacity to know. Von Hildebrand warns against a "certain familiarity with God, a false, clumsy complacency."[51] One should never be content with one's knowledge of God but should remain open to God's self-revelation.[52]

Then, based on what one knows of God, one ought to respond to God accordingly.[53] This response should not be a trivial loyalty as if one's relationship with the inscrutable God could be reduced to a few insignificant rules, or as if God were a ruthless tyrant who enjoys imposing arbitrary rules.[54] When confronted with God, the reverent man responds by seeking God's glorification. As a creature, he struggles to glorify God adequately and this drive of reverence leads to religion. Von Hildebrand writes that "reverence is the mother of . . . all religion."[55]

Von Hildebrand argues that the Catholic Liturgy, since it aims at God's glorification, develops the virtue of reverence in those who faithfully participate in it.[56] For example, the invitatory, recited at the beginning of evening prayer, "vividly presents before our mind . . . our absolute dependence on Him, the fact that we belong to Him."[57] Further, the Confiteor manifests one's need to acknowledge his sinful limitations before God: "Only after the appeal to God's mercy—the prayer Misereatur, the asking for forgiveness, and the Kyrie—does the Gloria follow, wherein once more the pure glorification of God is given expression."[58] Only after one recognizes his sinfulness before God can he offer a genuine response to God, a response of worship. Another example of how the liturgy fosters a right relationship with God is in the manner that God is addressed: "This feeling, that we only dare address God in Christ and through Christ, is one which is deeply opposed to all easy familiarity; it never allows us to forget the awe in which we must always make our approach to God."[59]

Man is distinguished from other earthly creatures by his capacity to show God reverence. Von Hildebrand writes, "Man alone can make a conscious response to God's endless glory."[60] Man cannot attain sanctification without reverence and man's ultimate dignity is found precisely in his ability to attentively adore and glorify God.[61]

Reverence is the foundation of morality: "Wherever we look, we see reverence to be the basis and at the same time an essential element of moral life and moral values. Without a fundamental attitude of reverence, no true love, no justice, no kindliness, no self-development, no purity, no truthfulness are possible."[62] Reverence is necessary for value perception, value response, virtue development, and in the strengthening of communities.

First, reverence is required for authentic contact with reality.[63] The reverent man "understands the dignity and nobility of being as such, the value which it already possesses in its opposition to mere nothingness."[64] The fact that things exist is a reality worthy of awe and contemplation. The reverent man further recognizes that being is created in a particular way: "there is a value inherent in every stone, in a drop of water, in a blade of grass, precisely as being, as an entity which possesses its own being, which is such and not otherwise. In contradistinction to a fantasy or a sheer semblance, being is something independent of the person considering it and withdrawn from that person's arbitrary will."[65]

The reverent man recognizes that the world is filled with things "important in themselves."[66] Each being possesses "its own consistency," a "standing on its own," and an "ultimate positivity."[67] Von Hildebrand writes, "The man who possesses reverence knows that . . . he must learn from being, not the other way around."[68] As much as the reverent man knows about the world, he remains vigilantly aware that more is yet to be revealed. Accordingly, he "leaves to being the space which it needs in order to unfold itself."[69]

His disposition toward the world is that of a discoverer continuously encountering new land and new features of previously recognized land.

The perception of values is significantly compromised in the absence of reverence. Von Hildebrand highlights pride and concupiscence as two particularly harmful forms of irreverence: "Only the man who can see beyond his subjective horizon and who, free from pride and concupiscence, does not always ask 'what is satisfying for me?' but who, leaving behind him all narrowness, abandons himself to that which is important in itself—the beautiful, the good—and subordinates himself to it, only he can become the bearer of moral values."[70] The prideful man approaches everything with a false familiarity, imagining "that he knows everything, that he sees through everything."[71]

In addition to the lack of openness exhibited by the prideful man, both the prideful and concupiscent fail to perceive reality because they are inordinately focused on goods serving selfish wants. An irreverent man "is the slave of his pride, of that cramping egoism which makes him a prisoner of himself, blind to values, and leads him to ask repeatedly 'will my prestige be increased, will my own glory by augmented?' Or he is a slave of concupiscence, one for whom everything in the world becomes only an occasion to serve his lust."[72] Such men fail "to leave to being the 'space' which it needs to unfold itself fully and in its proper mode."[73]

The inward focus of the prideful and concupiscent man leads him to a shallow existence: "To his insolent, conceited gaze, to his despotic approach, the world is sealed, silent, stripped of all mystery, deprived of all depth, flat and limited to one dimension. He stands in desolate emptiness, blind to all the values and secrets of being, circling endlessly around himself."[74] Von Hildebrand compares the primitive man who naively attributes everything to God with a modern irreverent man who "is completely absorbed by all that is secondary."[75] In the end he concludes, due to the shallow character of the irreverent man, that such a man, "in spite of all his knowledge, is far more 'stupid' than the most primitive savage possessing reverence."[76]

The values of creation do not compete with the awesomeness of God but rather manifest God's glory. Von Hildebrand explains that this relationship between created values and God is highlighted when one understands that every value is "a gift from God . . . bestowed upon us by His *charity*."[77] The fundamental meaning of creation is "to imitate and glorify God," to fulfill "the divine idea in its regard," to "radiate from God's being," and to reflect "His eternal light."[78] One's communion with God, therefore, reveals the nature and order of creation, and genuine contact with values helps one "to see everything *in conspectu Dei*."[79]

Reverence is also "an indispensable element of every response to value."[80] This is the case, first of all, because reverence is necessary for knowing values but also because reverence toward God serves "as a *causa exem-*

plaris, a model for our attitude toward all values."[81] By going outside of oneself and beyond oneself to understand and glorify God, one is disposed to do the same for God's creation. Further, by reverencing God one sees other values in their proper place and is able to respond accordingly. For example, by knowing that God alone is worthy of adoration, one understands that idolatry is not "a superabundance of love" toward created goods but rather a "diminution."[82] One honors and appreciates created goods only by understanding how those goods imitate and glorify God.

Since created values imitate God, reverence is man's appropriate stance before all values.[83] Each value has a meaning of its own that one must respect. Further, each value, as an imitation of God, communicates a message of God to man.[84] One's focus on created goods does not necessarily compete with focus on God. Von Hildebrand explains that one can "entertain a full contact with the object, to accord an ample response to its specific meaning, and yet at the same time to continue dwelling in the sacral atmosphere."[85] One's recognition that being presents an analogy of God establishes in man an "inward qualitative unity amidst the manifoldness of mundane objects and tasks."[86] This unity has implications for how von Hildebrand conceives of morality. Morality is less about fulfilling a "duty that goes against the heart's inclinations," and more focused on "the longing for union with each thing that possesses value and speaks to us of the glory of God, and especially with the longing for union with God Himself."[87]

One's adequate response to created values, in addition to being an indirect response to God, also expands man's capacity to respond to God. God uses created goods as "a path leading us to an ever-increasing unconditional surrender to Christ."[88] Von Hildebrand writes, "It is extremely important for us to profit by the moments when God draws us nearer to Him, when He allows us to be possessed by true values—and so loosens the fetters or our trivial system of petty self-protection and invites us to an act of ultimate audacity and freedom."[89] In this way, every value response thaws one's heart so that he may offer a more heartfelt response to God.[90]

The development of reverence through right relationship with God and awe for being also serves as the foundation for all virtues.[91] For example, reverence is the "presupposition for every true love,"[92] it confers "on our life a character of perfect simplicity,"[93] and is "the presupposition of purity."[94] The failure to perceive value and respond accordingly has the opposite effect: "The instant the person renounces this habitual response to a value and replaces it by indifference or even hostility to that value, becomes wholly dominated by pride or lust in his fundamental habitual attitude—his virtue is immediately lost. There is therefore no virtue which a man cannot lose."[95]

Von Hildebrand contrasts the reverent man, who respects creation as an imitation of God and therefore responds appropriately, with the prideful or concupiscent man, who sees the world merely as a means to his own practical aims.[96] The irreverent man does not take being "seriously for its own sake," and fails to see "its function of imitating God."[97] As a result, one approaches the world with increasing "technicalization and instrumentalization."[98] The world is perceived not as a gift from God full of mystery and depth and pointing toward God, but merely as fuel to attain one's personal ambitions or pleasure. The need for reverence toward the Creator and the gift of being has important implications in von Hildebrand's account of procreation.

D. THE PRIMARY END OF MARRIAGE

While von Hildebrand affirmed that procreation is the primary end of marriage, some of those who reviewed his work on *Marriage* argued that his emphasis on conjugal love undermined the importance of procreation in marriage.[99] Von Hildebrand argues that his account of conjugal love not only avoids undermining procreation's role in marriage but enhances that role. One can now examine this claim after understanding von Hildebrand's remarks on conjugal love, marriage, the conjugal act, the principle of superabundance, and the virtue of reverence. The criticisms concern issues of intentionality and procreation's primacy in marriage.

The 1917 Code of Canon Law, the active code while von Hildebrand wrote, states "The primary end of marriage is the procreation and education of children; the secondary [end] is mutual support and a remedy for conscupiscence."[100] Drawing on Thomas Aquinas' account of moral action, many theologians and canon lawyers of the early twentieth century interpreted this code to affirm that procreation should be the intention of marriage. Aquinas affirms that an action is determined formally by its end, that is, by "the object of the interior act of the will."[101] The end is first in the order of intention and last in the order of execution.[102] In other words, the end and the intention of the action are one and the same.[103] That which leads to an end, therefore, is chosen as a means to that end.[104] If the intention of the action is the end of the action and procreation is the primary end of marriage, then procreation should be the intention of marriage.

Von Hildebrand, while not denying that the intention and the end are often one in the same, explains that, in some actions, the fruit that occurs last in the order of execution flows superabundantly from a value response. In such actions, the value is the intention, that is, the value explains both why the action is performed and to what the moral agent gives his focused attention, even while the superabundant fruit is voluntarily willed.[105] For von Hildebrand, procreation is not the primary end in the sense of being the primary intention but is primary in some other way.

The question of how procreation is the primary end of marriage is not unique to von Hildebrand's account but is just as relevant for the teaching of Leo XIII, the 1917 Code of Canon Law, and Pius XI.[106] These authors certainly did not affirm the reduction of one's spouse to an instrumental means for attaining children. What then did they mean in affirming that procreation is the primary end of marriage? What is unique to von Hildebrand is the manner in which he surfaces the question by highlighting the importance of conjugal love and by identifying certain ways that procreation is not primary. Procreation is not primary as the main motivation for entering marriage, or as necessary to render a marriage valid or meaningful.[107] While von Hildebrand does not explicitly describe his meaning in affirming that procreation is the primary end of marriage, his analysis of reverence and procreation provides an implicit answer.

The German phrase that stands behind the phrase "primary end" is *primärer Zweck*. The term *Zweck* is commonly translated to English as function or purpose. Each of these two possible meanings has relevance for von Hildebrand's use of the term. Procreation has a functional relationship with the conjugal act in that the husband's sperm is released in relative proximity to his wife's ovaries. If an egg is released and a sperm unites with that egg, procreation will result. Von Hildebrand could mean that procreation is primary in the sense that, biologically speaking, procreation is the primary function of the conjugal act.

However, if procreation is primary as a functional consequence, then von Hildebrand certainly means more. The very biological structure of the human person is established by God and therefore communicates a word from God. Further, the conjugal act is not merely a biological process but a spiritual action which ought to be an actualization of conjugal love.

Zweck also could mean purpose. John Ford translates *Zweck* in this way when reviewing von Hildebrand's *Marriage*: "[Von Hildebrand] begins by distinguishing the primary meaning of marriage, which is conjugal love, from the primary purpose, which is procreation."[108] However, insofar as purpose means motivation for doing something, von Hildebrand affirms that the primary purpose of marriage is conjugal love and the mutual salvation of the spouses.[109] Since the salvation of souls is the universal purpose for all things, one might say that conjugal love is the primary purpose unique to both marriage and the conjugal act. Von Hildebrand does not seem to mean that both procreation and conjugal love are equally primary purposes. He affirms that one may enter marriage and express the conjugal act without being motivated by procreation but one should never express the conjugal act without the motivation of actualizing conjugal love.

Procreation is primary because the relationship between the conjugal act and procreation concerns, in a unique way, man's relationship with God. When von Hildebrand first affirms that procreation is the primary end of marriage, he adds, in the original German, a key adjective that gets dropped in the English translation; procreation is the "primärer Schöpfungszweck" (primary created end).[110] Although an infinite distance stands between the Creator and the creature, in procreation, God honors man by allowing man to cooperate in His Divine activity, something that man could never do without God. Procreation "draws the one who understands it *in conspectu Dei*—before the face of God."[111] Procreation is the Creator's loving invitation for creatures to participate in His Divine Power.[112] To ignore, deny, or appropriate the manner in which the Creator has ordered the conjugal act to procreation, is to irreverently desecrate this invitation. Procreation is primary to marriage and the conjugal act because man's disposition toward procreation impacts, at the most fundamental level, his relationship with God.[113]

E. THE ENHANCED ROLE OF PROCREATION IN MARRIAGE

By arguing that procreation is the primary end of marriage, von Hildebrand places his remarks within the tradition of the Catholic Church. However, he is not content to argue merely that his remarks on conjugal love are compatible with the affirmation that procreation is marriage's primary end. He makes the further claim that his remarks on conjugal love illuminate the link between marriage and procreation. He writes, "The distinction we have made between meaning and end, as well as the insight that marriage has a value of its own besides its sublime value as source of procreation, in no way diminishes the importance of the link between marriage and procreation; it rather enhances the link and places it in the right perspective."[114] His emphasis on conjugal love enhances procreation's role in marriage in two ways. First, reverence for conjugal love, marriage, and the conjugal act promote reverence for procreation. Second, discussion of conjugal love highlights that procreation is not merely biological but more importantly an overflow of love.

According to von Hildebrand, reverence for God transforms conjugal love, marriage and the conjugal act. Von Hildebrand argues that conjugal love is not based on selfish motives but genuine contact with the dignity of the beloved. In God, the lover sees the beloved as created by God in the image of God, redeemed by Jesus, and destined to eternal union with God.[115] In God, the lover discerns whether the beloved is the one with whom God has called him to enter marriage and whether marriage would promote the eternal welfare of both parties. Marriage is a divinely established community, raised to a Sacrament by Christ, indissoluble, and intended to serve as an image for Christ's love for the Church and the soul's eternal union with God.[116] In God, sexual intercourse is always a profound action which can be either the completion of marriage and actualization of conjugal love or an irreverent degradation and defilement of the moral agents, of conjugal love, of marriage, and of the conjugal act.[117] Reverence for God and the reverence before all created goods implied by reverence for God runs throughout von Hildebrand's account of conjugal love and marriage. His remarks on the divinely established connection between marriage and procreation simply complete the picture.[118]

If spouses are reverent toward God in their understanding of conjugal love, marriage and the conjugal act, then all the more so, they will be reverent in procreation. Von Hildebrand writes that the Creator "miraculously dignifies man to work with Him, to take part in His creative powers in the origination of a new man."[119] In reverence, spouses recognize that they participate in God's creative action and not the other way around. God alone, and not man, is Creator.[120]

Although God creates a human soul whenever sperm and egg unite, the spouses do not thereby become the primary agents of creation. God determined the means by which spouses share in His creative power. Further, God's contribution to new human life is by no means accidental as if life already was created by man and God simply adds the icing on the cake. God creates what He alone can create. He creates the core of man, namely, man's immortal soul.[121] Since God establishes the means of creation and since He alone creates the human soul, God remains the primary agent of creation: "the conjugal act of the spouses is incorporated into the creative act of God and acquires a serving function in relation to His act."[122]

Reverence, therefore, reveals the unique character of procreation. In procreation, spouses are called to acknowledge their position before the Creator and to stand in awe, reverence, and thanksgiving.[123] By recognizing their position before the Creator, spouses understand the great honor and mystery of procreation, namely that a creature participates in creating: "It is difficult to imagine a greater lack of reverence toward God than interfering with this mystery with desecrating hands."[124] In reverence, man leaves the domain of creating to God and only participates in that realm according to the means that God graciously has established.

Von Hildebrand's account of conjugal love further enhances procreation's role in marriage by highlighting that procreation, like all creation, is rooted in Divine Love. Reverence reveals that God's act of creation is an act of pure love and that everything man has is a Divine gift. God's Triune Love stands at the foundation of all things and overflows into His creation. God invites man to participate in His overflowing Love and one entryway into this Love is the vocation of marriage. God wills that couples enter marriage from the conviction that He has brought them together and that they will promote one another's eternal salvation through a fostering of mutual conjugal love. In procreation, spouses participate not only in the Creative Power of

God but further, through their loving expression of the conjugal act, embody God's Love and the creative power of Love: "As God's love is the creative principle in the universe, so love is everywhere creation, and there is a profound significance in the nexus—at once symbol and reality—whereby from the creative act—in which two become one flesh from love and in love—the new human being proceeds."[125]

Von Hildebrand finds great meaning in the fact that procreation results from an act of love. He frequently affirms that "God has entrusted the generation of a human being to the intimate union of man and wife who love each other in wedded love."[126] The link between love and procreation is not a coincidence or simply the reality of things, but rather a word of God to man communicating deep mysteries.[127] Despite the evil in the world, man's loving participation in God's Creative Power testifies that love and not sin is fundamental to existence. Emphasis on conjugal love does not detract from but increases the role of procreation in marriage by showing how God lifts man into His Divine and Loving activity.

Von Hildebrand's discussion of procreation works from the fruitfulness of God's love, through love in general, conjugal love and the conjugal act, to the fruitfulness of procreation. Procreation is an expression of God's fruitful Love—not the other way around. The link between conjugal love and procreation highlights how the conjugal act participates and manifests the fruitfulness of God's Love.[128]

F. SUMMARY

While von Hildebrand's remarks on conjugal love received almost universal praise, some early and more recent reviewers have critiqued von Hildebrand for falling short in his account of procreation. Their critique ranges from praising that von Hildebrand's remarks may be at odds with the Catholic tradition to saying that he simply neglects to give procreation a treatment that corresponds with his treatment of conjugal love. For his part, von Hildebrand is not content with arguing that his remarks on conjugal love do not directly contradict the tradition, or even to say that his remarks correspond with the tradition. He maintains that emphasis on conjugal enhances rather than diminishes procreation's role in marriage. He argues that one can recognize the link between procreation and marriage only after one understands marriage as a love union, the conjugal act as the consummation of marriage, reverence, and the principle of superabundance.

A unique development in the thought of von Hildebrand is his articulation of superabundant finality which plays a significant role in his analysis of procreation. He contrasts the principle of superabundance with instrumental finality. The key difference relates to the significance of the means. For instrumental finality, the significance of the means is reduced to its ability to attain the end. For superabundant finality, the means has independent significance regardless of whether the end results or not. Procreation is not an instrumental end of the conjugal act as if marriage, conjugal love, and the dignity of one's spouse could be reduced to their ability to promote procreation. Procreation is a superabundant fruit of the conjugal act. The conjugal act has meaning as the consummation of marriage and the actualization of conjugal love and procreation occasionally overflows as a superabundant fruit.

The way in which the conjugal act leads to procreation becomes clear in light of von Hildebrand's discussion of reverence. Man must recognize that he is a creature completely dependent and inferior to the Creator. Reverence requires that one allow God to reveal Himself to man and that man does not use God for his own relishes. The appropriate response to God is to seek His glory. Reverence is a basic requirement for moral inquiry. Openness to God leads to openness to God's creation and vice versa. Accordingly, conjugal love, marriage, and procreation are understood in relation to God.

While von Hildebrand argues that procreation is the primary end of marriage, his analysis of conjugal love raises questions about the meaning of this affirmation. Conjugal love, and not procreation, is the primary motivation for marriage and for expression of the conjugal act. Procreation is primary as the created end of the conjugal act. Although God alone is Creator, God honors spouses to participate in His Creative Power through the conjugal act. While God creates a human soul every time sperm and egg meet, He remains the primary agent of creation. He has established the means by which spouses can participate in creating and God alone creates the human soul. Spouses must leave the domain of creation to God alone and participate in that domain according to the means God generously has established. Procreation is primary because it deals with man's fundamental relationship with God as a creature before his Creator.

Von Hildebrand proposes that emphasis on conjugal love enhances rather than decreases procreation's role in marriage. He maintains that a reverent disposition toward conjugal love, marriage, and the conjugal act will enhance reverence for procreation. Conjugal love is not merely a subjective feeling that allows one to re-create the meaning of marriage and procreation. Marriage is a vocation to which God calls certain individuals in order to share with them His Divine Grace to work out their eternal salvation. The conjugal act is the consummation of marriage and the actualization of conjugal love. The conjugal act should be expressed only with God's sanction. If God is recognized throughout the development of conjugal love, entry into marriage and expression of the conjugal act, then He will more likely be recognized in one's disposition toward procreation. Emphasis on conjugal love highlights the honor of procreation and the manner in which God has ordained the conjugal act to lead to procreation.

Von Hildebrand works from the fruitfulness of God's Divine Love to the fruit of procreation. Accordingly, the fundamental reality is God's Love and the spiritual fruitfulness of conjugal love and the blessing of procreation should be understood in that light. The fact that procreation ought to flow from an act of love bears great significance. Procreation ought to manifest that the core reality of creation's existence is Love and not pride and concupiscence. That man is created in love points to his destiny of eternal participation in Triune Love.

Spouses, in expressing the conjugal act, must be attentive to two things: conjugal love's actualization and reverence for the God-established means of procreation. If spouses neglect one or the other, they fall into sin. If they seek a child to the neglect of conjugal love, they disregard the dignity of their spouse and the foundational reality that Love is the source of creation. If they neglect the connection between the conjugal act and procreation, they disregard their Creator who has honored the spouses with the means to participate in His Creative Powers. To avoid these two errors, von Hildebrand proposes that spouses should seek to actualize their conjugal love in the conjugal act while remaining aware of the manner in which God has linked this action with procreation.

Notes

1. *The Encyclical "Humanae Vitae,"* 29, italics in work cited.
2. *The Encyclical "Humanae Vitae,"* 29, see also 30 and *Man and Woman*, 93 and 97.
3. *Marriage*, 49, italics in work cited. Note that this section is a new addition to the 1942 English translation of *Die Ehe*. The section is not found in the original German text.
4. *Man and Woman*, 93-94; this sentence is repeated verbatim in the English translation of *The Encyclical "Humanae Vitae,"* 30; see also *Man and Woman*, 86 and *Purity*, 11.
5. *The Encyclical "Humanae Vitae,"* 31, italics in work cited; see also *The Encyclical "Humanae Vitae,"* 30, where von Hildebrand writes, "In the instrumental finality the *causa finalis* determines the *causa formalis*; in the superabundant the *causa formalis* differs from the *causa finalis*" (italics in work cited).
6. *Man and Woman*, 94.
7. *Man and Woman*, 93.
8. *Purity*, 11.
9. *Liturgy and Personality*, 6-7, italics in work cited.
10. He also employs the examples of knowledge and love to illustrate the principle of superabundance. He explains that while knowledge has value as the attainment of truth, it can also serve superabundant ends such as enabling man to act and to attain sanctification (*Man and Woman*, 93 and *The Encyclical "Humanae Vitae,"* 30). Similarly, the happiness resulting from loving another flows as a superabundant fruit (*The Encyclical "Humanae Vitae,"* 19).
11. See also von Hildebrand's discussion of moral consciousness in his *Christian Ethics* (New York: David McKay, 1953), 257-81.
12. Dietrich von Hildebrand, *Transformation in Christ*, trans. anonymous (San Francisco, CA: Ignatius Press, 1990), 54.
13. *Transformation in Christ*, 54; a few pages later he directs this insight to a critique of certain approaches to psychoanalysis: "Psychoanalysis is not only unfit to cure this morbid self-consciousness; it is even apt to increase the evil. For it incites its victims continually to dig for

the supposedly hidden motives of their thoughts instead of singly attending to the object" (p. 56).

14. *Transformation in Christ*, 54.
15. *Transformation in Christ*, 57.
16. *Transformation in Christ*, 59.
17. *The Encyclical "Humanae Vitae,"* 34-35.
18. *Purity*, 10-11.
19. *The Encyclical "Humanae Vitae,"* 45.
20. *Purity*, 13, italics in work cited; see also *Purity*, 10 and 12 and "Lambeth-Botschaft," 27.
21. *Purity*, 10.
22. *The Encyclical "Humanae Vitae,"* 31-32.
23. *The Encyclical "Humanae Vitae,"* 32, italics in work cited.
24. *The Encyclical "Humanae Vitae,"* 33, italics in work cited.
25. *The Encyclical "Humanae Vitae,"* 33; see also *Purity*, 11-12.
26. *Marriage*, 59-60.
27. This affirmation finds support in canon law: "Sterility neither impedes nor [renders illicit] marriage" (*Pio-Benedictine Code*, 1068, § 3, brackets in work cited; see also the 1983 *Code of Canon Law*, canon 1084, § 3). Augustine makes a similar observation in his work, *On the Good of Marriage*: "So strong is that bond of fellowship in married persons, that, although it be tied for the sake of begetting children, not even for the sake of begetting children is it loosed. For it is in a man's power to put away a wife that is barren, and marry one of whom to have children. And yet it is not allowed" (Augustine, *On the Good of Marriage*, trans. C. L. Cornish, in *Nicene and Post-Nicene Fathers*, vol. 3, ed. Philip Schaff [Peabody, Massachusetts: Hendrickson, 1994], 402; see also 400). One early reviewer of *Die Ehe* noted how von Hildebrand's discussion of conjugal love provides a unique framework for thinking about marriages not blessed with children (E. Schneider, review of *Die Ehe* by Dietrich von Hildebrand, *Theologie und Glaube* 21 [1929]: 813).
28. *Marriage*, 24.
29. *Marriage*, 24. While von Hildebrand compares a faithful and infertile marriage with a fertile and unfaithful marriage, he does not offer a similar comparison between two marriages that share the same depth of love but one of which is blessed with children and the other is not. Therefore, he leaves unanswered whether or not an infertile marriage, perhaps even one with a profound conjugal love, is a marriage lacking fulfillment without the fruit of children.
30. *Man and Woman*, 98; see also *The Encyclical "Humanae Vitae,"* 37 and Lambeth-Botschaft, 26-27.
31. *The Encyclical "Humanae Vitae,"* 37; von Hildebrand makes a similar observation in *Man and Woman*, 98-99.
32. *Marriage*, 26; von Hildebrand also writes that the desecration resulting from promiscuity "remains the same whether or not children result from this sinful union" (*Marriage*, 26).
33. *Marriage*, 23. Von Hildebrand is quoting Genesis 2:18; he does not indicate the translation he employs.
34. Von Hildebrand does not discuss Genesis 1:28 where God says, "Be fertile and multiply; fill the earth and subdue it" (*New American Bible*).
35. *Marriage*, 24.
36. Elizabeth Anscombe, *Intention* (Cambridge, Massachessetts, Harvard University Press, 1963), 37.
37. Anscombe, 37.
38. Anscombe, 37-38.
39. Dietrich von Hildebrand, *The Nature of Love*, trans. John F. Crosby (South Bend, Indiana: St. Augustine's Press, 2009), 46.
40. *Nature of Love*, 118-22.
41. *The Enyclical "Humanae Vitae,"* 43.
42. Dietrich von Hildebrand, *Liturgy and Personality*, newly revised, trans. anonymous (Baltimore, MD: Helicon Press, 1960).
43. Dietrich von Hildebrand and Alice von Hildebrand, *Art of Living*, rev. ed., trans. Alice von Hildebrand (Manchester, NH: Sophia Institute Press, 1994).

44. *Liturgy and Personality*, 38.
45. *Transformation in Christ*, 158.
46. *Transformation in Christ*, 158; see also *Liturgy and Personality*, 41.
47. *Transformation in Christ*, 158; see also *Liturgy and Personality*, 41 and 56.
48. *Liturgy and Personality*, 39.
49. *Liturgy and Personality*, 38.
50. *Liturgy and Personality*, 39.
51. *Liturgy and Personality*, 39.
52. *Liturgy and Personality*, 38.
53. *Liturgy and Personality*, 40.
54. *Liturgy and Personality*, 39.
55. *Liturgy and Personality*, 36; see also 38 and 39 and *Art of Living*, 11.
56. *Liturgy and Personality*, 40 and 43.
57. *Liturgy and Personality*, 41.
58. *Liturgy and Personality*, 56.
59. *Liturgy and Personality*, 42.
60. *Liturgy and Personality*, 10.
61. *Liturgy and Personality*, 10.
62. *Art of Living*, 10-11; see also 4 and 9.
63. *Ethics*, 232; see also *Liturgy and Personality*, 36 and *Art of Living*, 8.
64. *Art of Living*, 7; see also *Liturgy and Personality*, 36.
65. *Art of Living*, 7.
66. *Art of Living*, 4.
67. *Liturgy and Personality*, 36.
68. *Art of Living*, 7.
69. *Art of Living*, 7; von Hildebrand also explains that genuine contact with values in turn promotes further growth in reverence. The development of reverence and genuine contact with the world increase together (*Liturgy and Personality*, 37).
70. *Art of Living*, 4.
71. *Liturgy and Personality*, 37; see also *Art of Living*, 5.
72. *Art of Living*, 4; see also 6.
73. *Art of Living*, 6.
74. *Liturgy and Personality*, 37; see also *Art of Living*, 5.
75. *Liturgy and Personality*, 40; see also *Liturgy and Personality*, 39-40.
76. *Liturgy and Personality*, 40; see also 39.
77. *Transformation in Christ*, 96, italics in work cited.
78. *Liturgy and Personality*, 9; see also 37 and 45.
79. *Transformation in Christ*, 498.
80. *Liturgy and Personality*, 37; see also *Liturgy and Personality*, 47 and *Art of Living*, 8.
81. *Liturgy and Personality*, 43.
82. *Marriage*, 38-39.
83. *Liturgy and Personality*, 37.
84. Von Hildebrand proposes that "the higher a good and the more directly it is in its own nature connected with God, the more it glorifies God directly" (*Marriage*, 42).
85. *Transformation in Christ*, 98.
86. *Transformation in Christ*, 98.
87. *Liturgy and Personality*, 53; von Hildebrand critiques Kant for failing to recognize the ethical significance of affective responses (*Ethics*, 344-45).
88. *Transformation in Christ*, 496.
89. *Transformation in Christ*, 497.
90. *Transformation in Christ*, 496.
91. *Liturgy and Personality*, 36 and *Purity*, 35; von Hildebrand gives further discussion to the topic of virtues in his 1952 work on *Ethics*, 342-46 and 357-78. In particular, see *Ethics*, 345-46, where von Hildebrand writes, "The sphere of virtues also has been fully ignored by Kant, and most of the ethicians since Kant have stepped into the same path. In contradistinction to this consideration of virtues, the ethics of antiquity, as well as the ethics of St. Augustine and

St. Thomas, have attributed to virtues a great moral significance" (see also *Ethics*, 343). Von Hildebrand also proposes that reverence is the foundation of community (*Art of Living*, 10).

92. *Art of Living*, 9; see also *Liturgy and Personality*, 39, where von Hildebrand proposes that reverence is the foundation for faith, hope, and love.

93. *Transformation in Christ*, 98.

94. *Art of Living*, 10.

95. *Purity*, 36.

96. *Liturgy and Personality*, 38 and *Art of Living*, 7.

97. *Liturgy and Personality*, 45; see also 39.

98. *Liturgy and Personality*, 39.

99. Von Hildebrand writes that procreation is the primary end of marriage in his works on *Marriage* (v, vi, 4, 21, 25), *Man and Woman* (p. 81), and *The Encyclical "Humanae Vitae"* (p. 35). Those who question whether von Hildebrand in fact maintains the primary of procreation include Bernard Lonergan, review of *Marriage*, by Dietrich von Hildebrand, in *Shorter Papers*, vol. 20 of *Collected Works of Bernard Lonergan*, ed. Frederick Crowe and Robert Doran (Toronto: University of Toronto Press, 2007), 155; John C. Ford, review of *Marriage*, by Dietrich von Hildebrand, *Thought* 17 (September 1942): 544-45; Arjonillo, 302; and Michael Gierens, review of *Die Ehe*, by Dietrich von Hildebrand, *Stimmen der Zeit* 119 (1930): 386.

100. *The 1917 Pio-Benedictine Code of Canon Law*, trans. Edward N. Peters (San Francisco, CA: Ignatius Press, 2001), Canon 1013, §1, brackets in work cited.

101. Thomas Aquinas, *Treatise on Happiness*, trans. John A. Oesterle (Notre Dame, IN: University of Notre Dame Press, 1964), II-I, Q. 18, a. 6, 168; see also Q. 1, a. 3.

102. Aquinas, II-I, Q. 1, a. 4.

103. See John C. Ford, review of *Marriage*, by Dietrich von Hildebrand, *Thought* 17 (September 1942): 544-45.

104. Aquinas, II-I, Q. 12, a. 4, reply 3.

105. Although those critiquing von Hildebrand draw on Thomistic language, Aquinas anticipates von Hildebrand's insight about superabundant finality in important ways. Von Hildebrand's notion of superabundance has strong affinity to Aquinas's notion of consequences that relates to the essence of an action (Aquinas, II-I, Q. 20, a. 5). Aquinas also notes that some things while serving as a means to end have goodness in themselves apart from the end they serve (Aquinas, II-I, Q. 20, a. 3; II-I, Q. 16, a. 3, reply 2). For further comparison of von Hildebrand's principle of superabundance and Aquinas' account of ends, see Alice von Hildebrand, "Aristotle: The Philosopher," *Logos* 8, 3 (Summer 2005): 112-22. For a critique of von Hildebrand's remarks on this topic in relation to the final good of happiness, see Michael Waldstein, "Dietrich von Hildebrand and St. Thomas Aquinas on Goodness and Happiness,"*Nova et Vetera* 1, 2 (2003): 403-64.

106. See, for example, John Ford's attempt to answer the question, how is procreation primary? Ford affirms that procreation is primary because "procreation 'is more important, and more fundamental' (*Marriage Questions*, 128-30). He states that the "secondary ends presuppose, that is, depend on or are subordinate to the primary ends in a sense in which the primary ends do not presuppose or depend on the secondary ends. In a word the primary ends are more fundamental" (*Marriage Questions*, 131). He also concludes that the other rights of marriage seem ordered to procreation (*Marriage Questions*, 135). Ford does not explain, however, what he means by more important, more fundamental, greater dependence or the implications of reducing marriage to the disposal of rights.

107. Von Hildebrand contends "that the term 'end' is used in traditional philosophy in a very loose sense; we should even say in an analogous sense. And as soon as an analogous term is understood as univocal, it leads to ambiguities. Thus, it remains necessary to shed light on the special type of finality which underlies the definition of procreation as the primary end of marriage" (*Man and Woman*, 85). While von Hildebrand shows that procreation is not primary as motivation or as required for a valid marriage, he affirms that such distinctions help to show how procreation is primary. In the process, however, von Hildebrand expresses concern that readers will neglect his analysis because of the impression that he is denying the traditional affirmation that procreation is primary (*Man and Woman*, 85-86).

108. Ford, review of *Marriage*, 544. Ford's use of "purpose" is particularly peculiar here since Ford is reviewing the English translation of *Die Ehe*, in which *Zweck* is consistently translated as "end" and not "purpose." Bruehl also uses purpose in his review of *Marriage*, 234. Although I am not certain why Ford and Bruehl use purpose in relation to von Hildebrand's discussion of procreation, possible sources include the Vatican's English translation of Pius XI's *Casti connubii* ("On Christian Marriage") or George Sayer's English translation of Herbert Doms's *Vom Sinn und Zweck der Ehe* ("The Meaning of Marriage"). Pius XI's, *On Christian Marriage*, refers to procreation as the purpose of marriage (Pius XI, *On Christian Marriage*, trans. anonymous [Boston, MA: St. Paul Editions, neither the publication date nor the translation are listed; the cover states, "Official Vatican Text"], paragraph numbers 54 and 80; *AAS* 22 (1930): 559 and 570.The introduction to Doms' *The Meaning of Marriage* reads, "It was this which prompted Dietrich von Hildebrand to distinguish between the *meaning* and the *purpose* of marriage and of physical union, and to specify community in love as the 'meaning'" (Herbert Doms, *The Meaning of Marriage*, trans. George Sayer [London: Sheed and Ward, 1939], xvi, italics in work cited).

109. For the background of my use of the phrase "purpose," see Francis Slade, "Ends and Purposes," in *Final Causality in Nature and Human Affairs*, ed. Richard F. Hassing (Washington, D.C.: The Catholic University of America, 1997), 83-84.

110. *Die Ehe*, 7, my translation; see *Marriage*, 4, where this phrase is translated as "primary *end*" (italics in work cited).

111. *The Encyclical "Humanae Vitae,"* 46.

112. *Marriage*, 23 and 52; "Lambeth-Botschaft," 21; *Man and Woman*, 93; *The Encyclical "Humanae Vitae,"* 29, 37, and 40.

113. Von Hildebrand affirms the centrality of procreation in marriage in his earlier work on *Marriage*. He includes in his summary of this work that in marriage "two persons are one in one flesh and have been allowed to participate in the creation of a new human being by God" (p. 52; see also "Lambeth-Botschaft," 21-22). Similarly, von Hildebrand affirms in *The Encyclical "Humanae Vitae,"* "To the sublime link between marriage and procreation Christ's words on the marriage bond also apply: 'What God has joined together, let no man put asunder'" (p. 36).

114. *The Encyclical "Humanae Vitae,"* 35; see also *The Encyclical "Humanae Vitae,"* 29 and *Man and Woman*, 93 and 97.

115. For von Hildebrand's discussion of the connection between reverence and recognizing the dignity of the human person see *Marriage*, 9 and 36-37, and *Art of Living*, 9. For von Hildebrand's discussion of the connection between reverence and other features of conjugal love, see, *Marriage*, 24, 35, 38, and 62.

116. For von Hildebrand's discussion of the connection between reverence and marriage see, *Marriage*, 29-31, 34, 41-47, 53, 60, and 62-64. See also *Purity*, 40.

117. For von Hildebrand's discussion of the connection between reverence and the conjugal act see, *Purity*, 10, 22, 23, 40-44, 46, 51, and 72-73, *Man and Woman*, 23 and 88-92, and *The Encyclical "Humanae Vitae,"* 9.

118. Von Hildebrand affirms that one can understand the link between procreation and both spousal love and the conjugal act only after one recognizes the link between spousal love and both marriage and the conjugal act (*Purity*, 15, *Man and Woman*, 91, and *The Encyclical "Humanae Vitae,"* 29).

119. "Lambeth-Botschaft," 21, my translation. The original German reads: "In wunderbarer Weise hat Gott den Menschen gewürdigt, an dem Entstehen neuer Menschen—mit unsterblichen, für die Ewigkeit bestimmten Seelen—mitzuwirken, an Seiner Schöpferkraft teilzuhaben." Von Hildebrand also refers to procreation as man's cooperation in divine creativity at *Marriage*, 23 and 52; *Man and Woman*, 93; and *The Encyclical "Humanae Vitae,"* 29 and 37; see also *Purity*, 14, where von Hildebrand speaks of the "creative significance" of the conjugal act.

120. *The Encyclical "Humanae Vitae,"* 35, 40, 47, and 87; *Man and Woman*, 98; and "Lambeth-Botschaft," 28.

121. *The Encyclical "Humanae Vitae,"* 36; see also footnote on *Purity*, 15.

122. *The Encyclical "Humanae Vitae,"* 37.

123. *The Encyclical "Humanae Vitae,"* 29; see von Hildebrand's reflections on gratitude in *Art of Living*, 103-39.

124. *Marriage*, 23.

125. *Purity*, 14-15; see also *Marriage*, 25. For von Hildebrand's discussion of the spiritual fruitfulness of the conjugal act, see *Marriage*, 39-40.

126. *The Encyclical "Humanae Vitae,"* 40; see also *Marriage*, 22; "Lambeth-Botschaft," 21; *Man and Woman*, 93; *The Encyclical "Humanae Vitae,"* xi, 29, and 35.

127. See *Marriage*, 4, *Man and Woman*, 85, and *The Encyclical "Humanae Vitae,"* xi, xiv, and 29. Von Hildebrand highlights the mysterious link between the conjugal act and procreation at *Purity*, 14 and 41 and the relationship between conjugal love and procreation at *Marriage*, 21 and 23; *Man and Woman*, 93; *The Encyclical "Humanae Vitae,"* 37, 41, and 46; and *Art of Living*, 10.

128. John Paul II makes a similar claim to that of von Hildebrand when he writes, "the family must go back to the 'beginning' of God's creative act, if it is to attain self-knowledge and self-realization in accordance with the inner truth not only of what it is but also of what it does in history. And since in God's plan it has been established as an 'intimate community of life and love,' the family has the mission to become more and more what it is, that is to say, a community of life and love, in an effort that will find fulfillment, as will everything created and redeemed, in the Kingdom of God. Looking at it in such a way as to reach its very roots, we must say that the essence and role of the family are in the final analysis specified by love. Hence the family has *the mission to guard, reveal and communicate love*, and this is a living reflection of and a real sharing in God's love for humanity and the love of Christ the Lord for the Church His bride. . . . Thus, with love as its point of departure and making constant reference to it, the recent Synod emphasized four general tasks for the family:

1) forming a community of persons;
2) serving life;
3) participating in the development of society;
4) sharing in the life and mission of the Church" (*Familiaris Consortio*, section 17, paragraphs 2-4, 32-33, italics in work cited).

Chapter Five

The Rhythm Method

The 1960s provide von Hildebrand a unique chance to clarify the relationship between conjugal love and procreation. Notions of free love, influential theories of overpopulation, and the publication of *Humanae vitae* raise a number of questions about the nature of the conjugal act and procreation. In his 1966 work, *Man and Woman*, von Hildebrand summarizes his earlier remarks in *Marriage* and addresses the question of overpopulation. Then, in his 1969 work, *The Encyclical "Humanae Vitae,"* he defends *Humanae vitae*'s support of the rhythm method.[1] Von Hildebrand's defense of the rhythm method is consistent with his earlier discussions found in *Purity* and "Lambeth-Botschaft." Nonetheless, since von Hildebrand writes the later works amid conversation about overpopulation, one does well to note the influence (or lack thereof) of that context on this thought.

A. OVERPOPULATION

Von Hildebrand concludes his work, *Man and Woman*, with a chapter titled "Marriage and Overpopulation." He does not question theories of overpopulation but accepts that overpopulation is a major issue. He explains that overpopulation has changed the general public's view of conception, pregnancy, childbirth, and raising children: "until now, a nation has always considered an increase in population as a great common good—a consideration which once assumed a unique character and a higher significance in the elect people of Israel—today the increase of population threatens to become a calamity."[2]

Von Hildebrand describes overpopulation not merely in terms of perspectives common in his day but as a perspective he shares: "there is little doubt that it is imperative to do something against the threat of overpopulation."[3] Nonetheless, his emphasis is not to prove or disprove overpopulation or even to solve the problem of overpopulation but rather to take the context of his day as an opportunity to re-affirm and clarify the meaning of marriage.[4]

For von Hildebrand, the "threat of overpopulation" raises a number of questions about marriage and procreation:

> What kind of means are morally unobjectionable in order to meet this threat? Does the fact that the avoidance of conception becomes to a large extent an imperative obligation for the sake of the common good of humanity imply that far fewer people should get married? Does it deprive marriage of its meaning? Or does it at least undermine the *raison d'être* of the bodily union of the spouses? Does it drive us to either artificial birth control or abstinence?[5]

In this second to last paragraph of the same article, von Hildebrand raises similar questions and then concludes, "Certainly the answers to all these questions must be in the negative."[6] Theories of overpopulation do not alter von Hildebrand's position on the meaning of both marriage and the conjugal act. They do, however, provide him an opportunity to discuss in more detail the moral use of the rhythm method.

B. THE RHYTHM METHOD

Von Hildebrand discusses the rhythm method in response to two documents issued by Christian leaders. In the first instance, he writes a short response article to the 1930 Lambeth Conference. Nearly forty years later, von Hildebrand writes a defense of Pope Paul VI's, *Humanae vitae*. While von Hildebrand's position does not change, his focus does. Whereas in the earlier article his focus was to show why use of the rhythm method is acceptable, in the latter work he seeks to demonstrate why children are a gift and not a burden, why the rhythm method is natural, and whether or not the abstinence involved in the rhythm method is a reasonable sacrifice for spouses.

In his 1930 article, "Lambeth-Botschaft," von Hildebrand gives the impression that Catholic leaders have approved the temporary avoidance of children through use of the rhythm method. Without citing the statement to which he is referring, he writes, "the holy Penitentiary even explains that spouses who want to avoid descendents for a time out of morally legitimate grounds are allowed to select days with facultative sterility for sexual union."[7] John Noonan's historical summary of church teaching concerning use of infertile periods to avoid conception indicates that the most relevant Penitentiary statement to date would have been an 1880 decision dealing with "onanism."[8] The statement declares that confessors should leave spouses undisturbed who are using the rhythm method to avoid conception and that confessors could subtly point spouses toward temporary abstinence during fertile periods if other measures to prevent "onanism" have failed.[9]

The question about use of the rhythm method was posed again to the Penitentiary one year after von Hildebrand's "Lambeth-Botschaft" article. However, this statement simply re-affirmed the 1880 decision.[10] Noonan indicates that *general* use of sterile periods to avoid conception did not receive official Roman approval until Pius XII's 1951 address to the Italian Catholic Society of Midwives: "For the first time rhythm was referred to by Roman authority not as an alternative to be cautiously proffered to onanists, but as a method open to all Christian couples."[11]

While the 1880 decision does not affirm general use of the rhythm method to avoid procreation, neither does the document deny such a position.[12] Von Hildebrand sees in the 1880 statement recognition that recourse to infertile periods can be morally justified in certain situations. Within that framework, he formulates his own conclusions about general use of the rhythm method. Therefore, although von Hildebrand begins his discussion of the rhythm method with reference to Roman authority, his remarks on the rhythm method precede official Roman approval by some twenty years.

Von Hildebrand is able to affirm use of the rhythm method in part because of the framework he established in his works on *Purity* and *Marriage*. He asserts that conjugal love is the primary motivation for marriage. The conjugal act retains significance in addition to procreation, namely, as the actualization of conjugal love and the consummation of marriage. Infertile marriages remain valid and meaningful as an actualization of conjugal love. The domain of creating belongs uniquely to God. Spouses should not alter the means by which God allows them to cooperate in His creative power but since the conjugal act is a free, spiritual act, spouses may choose when to express the conjugal act. Spousal use of the rhythm method is acceptable because spouses maintain reverence for the means God has established for procreation and the conjugal act remains meaningful as the actualization of conjugal love and the consummation of marriage.[13]

In his defense of *Humanae vitae*, von Hildebrand further proposes that spouses deliberately may avoid the conception of a child: "it is definitely allowed *expressly* to avoid conception when the conjugal act takes place *only* in the *God-given* infertile time."[14] Von Hildebrand acknowledges that the direct avoidance of children found in use of the rhythm method involves a kind of separation between the conjugal act and the end of procreation.[15] He maintains, however, that this is an acceptable separation insofar as the "separation" is established by God.

C. THE GOOD OF CHILDREN

The spouses' normative disposition should be one that voluntary wants and seeks procreation in the conjugal act.[16] In "Lambeth-Botschaft," he affirms that spouses should avoid conception through use of the rhythm method only "out of morally legitimate grounds" or "out of serious grounds."[17] He confirms this position in his defense of *Humanae vitae* when he asserts that conception should be avoided for "good and valid reasons" or "serious reasons."[18] He does not explain what "good," "valid," or "serious" reasons would be but he repeatedly mentions the qualification indicating that voluntarily wanting children should be spouses' default disposition.

Despite his affirmation that spouses should prevent conception only for serious reasons, von Hildebrand writes little to nothing about the responsibility of parents to have children or the joy and fulfillment of having children. His emphasis on the good of children is implied but not explicitly highlighted in his published writings until he writes *The Nature of Love* in 1971. In this latter work, when he discusses objective goods for the person, he highlights children as a clear and dramatic example of an objective good mutually experienced.[19] He speaks of children being entrusted by God to their parents.[20] Children are a sign of hope, and an embodiment of purity and human vulnerability.[21] Von Hildebrand intended to develop this theme of the good of children more fully at a later time. Twice in *The Nature of Love*, he states that he will discuss in greater detail in a second volume, a volume that was never published, the love of parents for their children and the love of children for their parents.[22] Von Hildebrand's analysis of conjugal love, marriage, and the conjugal act certainly provides a fertile lens through which to see the good of children. One can see the fruitfulness of von Hildebrand's framework by integrating his remarks with more complete accounts of the responsibility of parents to have children and the gift of children, such as Pius XII's "Apostolate of the Midwife," *Gaudium et spes*, *Humanae vitae*, *Familiaris consortio*, and Janet Smith's *Humanae Vitae: A Generation Later*.

Procreation's role in marriage is not merely a legal obligation to which other goods are subordinate. Rather, as Pius XII states, to procreate and educate children "is a high and noble office (*Alto e nobile ufficio!*)" which belongs specifically to spouses.[23] Similarly, the Council Fathers write in *Gaudium et spes* about the "lofty role" of fathers and mothers.[24] This lofty role has a central place in marriage: "Without intending to underestimate the other ends of marriage, it must be said that true married love and the whole structure of family life which results from it is directed to disposing the spouses to cooperate valiantly with the love of the Creator and Saviour, who through them will increase and enrich his family from day to day."[25]

Janet Smith, who has done significant work on the encyclical *Humanae vitae* and on procreation's role in marriage, highlights the role or mission of spouses to procreate and educate children. She argues that emphasis on this mission in *Humanae vitae* has been neglected in part because of an inadequate translation of the term *munus*. Paul VI opens *Humanae vitae* speaking of "the most serious duty [*munus*] of transmitting human life."[26] Smith notes that this opening phrase connects *Humanae vitae* with a similar observation made near the end of *Gaudium et spes*' section on marriage: "Let all be convinced that human life and [the *munus* of] its transmission are realities whose meaning is not limited by the horizons of this life only; their true evaluation and full meaning can only be understood in reference to man's eternal destiny."[27]

Smith explains that, in the opening phrase of *Humanae vitae*, the term *munus* is often translated in English as "duty." She argues that this translation fails to communicate the positive character of *munus*: "The chief problem with the translation 'duty' is that for many modern English-speaking people the word has a negative sense. A duty is often thought of as something that one ought to do and something that one often is reluctant to do . . . a *munus* is something that one is honored and, in a sense, privileged to have."[28] According to Smith, "*Munera* are conferred by one superior in power on another; . . . *Munera* are not man-made but God-given."[29] The *munus* of parenting refers to a "special assignment" or "service to God."[30] Smith proposes that the opening phrase of *Humanae vitae* points not to a duty but to "the extremely important [*gravissimum*] mission [*munus*] of transmitting human life."[31]

The God-given mission of parenting highlights the unique gift of procreation. The loving Creator allows His creatures to participate in His loving and creative power and entrusts them with the important task of transmitting and caring for human life. John Paul II, who shares von Hildebrand's phenomenological background and attentiveness to conjugal love, affirms that God calls spouses "to a special sharing in His love and in His power as Creator and Father, through their free and responsible cooperation in transmitting the gift of human life."[32] Similarly, the Council Fathers describe children both as the "crowning glory" and "supreme gift" of marriage and married love.[33] John Paul II adds "that human life, even if weak and suffering, is always a splendid gift of God's goodness."[34]

The God-given mission of procreating and educating children is not an arbitrary honor and responsibility but rather a mission that corresponds with the vocation of marriage and therefore contributes to the salvation of both children and parents. The mission contributes to the children's salvation insofar as parents raise the children in the faith. John Paul II writes, "A vivid and attentive awareness of the mission that they have received with the sacrament of marriage will help Christian parents to place themselves at the service of their children's education with great serenity and trustfulness, and also with a sense of responsibility before God, who calls them and gives them the mission of building up the Church in their children."[35]

In return, as *Gaudium et spes* affirms, children "greatly contribute to the good of the parents."[36] John Paul II adds, "Family communion can only be preserved and perfected through a great spirit of sacrifice. It requires, in fact, a ready and generous openness of each and all to understanding, to forbearance, to pardon, to reconciliation."[37] In other words, as Janet Smith explains, having children "helps parents mature and acquire many of the virtues they need to be fully human and fully Christian."[38]

Since God gives the mission of procreating and educating children to spouses, the discernment of family size falls primarily on them.[39] The role of the state, therefore, is not to determine family size but to support families. Pius XI writes that when wages and charity do not allow parents to care for children, then "it is the duty of the public authority to supply for the insufficient forces of individual effort, particularly in a matter which is of such importance to the common weal."[40] John Paul II condemns those governments that instead of supporting families seek to limit the freedom of spouses to determine family size: "violence applied by such authorities in favor of contraception or, still worse, of sterilization and procured abortion, must be altogether condemned and forcefully rejected. Likewise to be denounced as gravely unjust are cases where . . . economic help given for the advancement of peoples is made conditional on programs of contraception, sterilization and procured abortion."[41]

Paul VI asserts that spouses must be aware of their important mission and they must discern how to execute that office responsibly.[42] He explains that this discernment should be done in relation to God and His created order: "the mission [*munere*] of responsible parenthood requires that spouses recognize their duties [*officia*] toward God, toward themselves, toward the family, and toward human society."[43] Accordingly, spouses should not choose arbitrarily how parenthood will be exercised in their marriage. On the contrary, they must seek to do God's will in accordance with the nature of marriage and with the guidance of the Church.[44]

Pius XII asserts that willingness to accept children lovingly is necessary but not sufficient for the moral use of the rhythm method: "the moral licitness of such conduct on the part of the couple would have to be approved or denied according as to whether or not the intention of observing those periods constantly was based on sufficient and secure moral grounds."[45] In other words, one does not do enough to show that use of the rhythm method is not irreverent or destructive of human life, one also must recognize the mission of procreating and educating children and seek to postpone the responsibilities of that mission only in the presence of serious reasons.

The Council Fathers and Paul VI acknowledge that spouses may have serious reasons for postponing children. *Gaudium et spes* states that those who are married "can sometimes find themselves in a position where the number of children cannot be increased, at least for the time being."[46] Paul VI adds that responsible parenthood includes those spouses who "for serious reasons [*seriis causis*] and with due respect for moral precepts, decide not to have another child for either a definite or an indefinite amount of time."[47]

Pius XII identifies some reasons that would justify use of the rhythm method to prevent conception:

> There are serious motives, such as those often mentioned in the so-called medical, eugenic, economic, and social 'indication,' that can exempt for a long time, perhaps even the whole duration of the marriage, from the positive and obligatory carrying out of the act. From this it follows that observing the non-fertile periods alone can be lawful only under a moral aspect. Under the conditions mentioned it really is so.[48]

Paul VI highlights four categories to consider in the discernment of family size: "physical, economic, psychological, and social conditions."[49] Despite listing relevant categories for consideration, Pius XII and Paul VI do not provide detailed application of these principles. Such application is ultimately left to spouses and their confessors.

One should note that the Council Fathers and Paul VI honor those spouses who responsibly procreate and educate a large number of children. The Council Fathers state,

> Whenever Christian spouses in a spirit of sacrifice and trust in divine providence carry out their duties of procreation with generous human and Christian responsibility, they glorify the Creator and perfect themselves in Christ. Among the married couples who thus fulfill their God-given mission, special mention should be made of those who after prudent reflection and common decision courageously undertake the proper upbringing of a large number of children.[50]

Similarly, Paul VI adds, "responsible parenthood is exercised by those who, guided by prudent consideration and generosity, elect to accept many children."[51] These affirmations honor spouses not merely because they have large families but because they have large families in a spirit of sacrifice, trust, prudence, and responsibility.[52]

Von Hildebrand discusses the vocation of marriage and asserts that marriage is a path to holiness. This insight is complemented by Pius XII, the Council Fathers, Paul VI and John Paul II's discussion of the mission of parenting. A significant aspect of God's call for spouses to attain holiness comes through the procreation and education of children. In this regard, spouses should buttress the reverence that von Hildebrand emphasizes with themes that he does not highlight in reference to procreation, namely, the prudence and generosity necessary to discern family size.

At the same time, von Hildebrand's emphasis on conjugal love prevents a possible misreading of the important mission of parenting. Marriage should not be reduced to procreation. A valid sacramental marriage does not require the gift of a child but rather procreation flows as the superabundant fruit of marriage. The fruit of procreation is not the foundation from which to understand the spiritual fruit of conjugal love and the fruitful love of God. Rather, God's overflowing love is the foundation for the fruit of conjugal love, which in turn is the foundation for procreation.

Spouses should voluntarily want children but may for serious reasons postpone the conception of a child. At this point, a further question needs to be asked: by what means may spouses postpone conception? When explaining the crucial distinction between recourse to infertile periods and employment of artificial birth control, Paul VI writes, "In the first, the spouses legitimately use a faculty that is given by nature; in the second case, the spouses impede the order of generation [*ordo generationis*] from completing its own natural processes."[53] Von Hildebrand defends Paul VI's claim by focusing on and clarifying the term "nature."[54] In particular, von Hildebrand seeks to demonstrate why human persons may intervene in certain areas of God's created order but not in others. He frames the question by distinguishing between two understandings of the term "nature."

D. NATURE

Nature can mean "the purely factual order of creation, especially material and biological creation" or "the essence of profoundly significant relations endowed with a high value."[55] As an example of the "purely factual," von Hildebrand describes the nine month period of pregnancy. He proposes that this period of time could just as easily be eight or ten months. He then affirms that a doctor may deliver a baby at eight months if the life of the baby or mother requires an early delivery. Any moral significance attributed to the nine month period of pregnancy comes not from the fact that pregnancy usually takes nine months but from some other foundation, such as the fact that healthy development of the baby usually takes about nine months.[56]

As an example of a deeply meaningful relation, von Hildebrand discusses "the fact that love brings happiness."[57] While human persons have the freedom to pursue happiness without taking the path of love, such a pursuit will reward individuals with only a shallow and fleeting happiness. Man is not truly fulfilled unless he loves. This relationship between love and happiness relates to the nature of both love and human happiness. This deeply ingrained relationship also points to God's Love which stands at the foundation and fulfillment of all creation. The call to love speaks not merely of a biological ordering of things but a call to respect and respond to the value of persons.

Concerning when human persons may morally manipulate the order of things, von Hildebrand writes that "nature" in the first sense,

> does not constitute something in which man ought not to intervene when there are reasonable grounds for seeking a change (in some circumstances he is even *obliged* to intervene). But intervention in nature in the second sense, where meaning and value are grounded in the essence of a thing, has a completely different character. For this nature contains in its very meaning and value a unique message from God and calls upon us to respect it.[58]

The second kind of nature cannot be manipulated because the thing under consideration not only relates to the essence of something created, but involves some deep value. He writes, "The *essential* difference between the two concepts of nature is not that in the one case we are confronted with an intelligible necessity fact and in the other with a mere empirical fact, but rather that in the one relations are deeply meaningful and possess a high *value*, and in the other they are only factual."[59]

Von Hildebrand's three-page discussion of nature provides a nice distinction for thinking about natural law and the limits of human intervention in God's created order. Some things have a high value and meaning and other things with less significance may be manipulated when circumstances merit intervention. He does not claim to offer categories that would allow one to discern, in every situation or even in most situations, when one may intervene in God's created order and when one should not intervene. In this, his account certainly does not answer the many questions raised about natural law following the publication of *Humanae vitae*.[60] He offers a modest contribution, nonetheless, by highlighting one important consideration in the discernment of when one should and should not intervene in God's created order, namely, the value of the thing involved.

For von Hildebrand, the link between the conjugal act and procreation involves nature in the second sense of the term. He writes, "it is not a merely factual or exclusively biological connection but rather a great and sublime mystery that God has entrusted the generation of a human being to the intimate union of man and wife who love each other in wedded love and who in becoming 'two in one flesh' participate in the creative act of God."[61] Here, von Hildebrand means mystery in the sense that the content is infinite, not in the sense that we cannot know anything about the connection. The God-established link between the conjugal act and procreation is profound because the connection reveals how creation flows superabundantly from the Creator's Triune Love. As with all instances where nature involves a deeply significant relation, one should not alter God's established order: "Any violence done to these [connections] is particularly presumptuous on the part of man the creature. It is the usurpation of a right which man does not possess; it reflects a desire to play the role of God and Providence."[62]

Von Hildebrand's affirmation about the deep connection between the conjugal act and procreation raises questions for spousal use of the rhythm method with the intention of postponing pregnancy. Does not the rhythm method involve a separation between the conjugal act and procreation? Von Hildebrand proposes that the rhythm method is an acceptable "separation" because it is established by God:

> In the intention itself of avoiding another child for serious reasons there is not the least trace of irreverence toward the mysterious fact that God has entrusted the birth of a person to the spousal love union. We see that only during relatively brief intervals has God Himself linked the conjugal act to the creation of a man. . . . The fact that conception is restricted to a short time implies a word of God. It not only confirms that the bodily union of the spouses has a meaning and value in itself apart from procreation, but it also leaves open the possibility of avoiding conception if this is desirable for serious reasons.[63]

Spouses, for serious reasons, may be attentive to their God-given fertility and seek to avoid conception by choosing when to express the conjugal act. In other words, God establishes the means by which humanity can participate in His creative powers even while "the moment of when to enter this domain is a choice open to men in marriage."[64]

The so-called separation refers to a separation of intention and consequence not a separation of the God-established link between the conjugal act and procreation. A separation of intention occurs in that spouses will to avoid conception insofar as they both have serious reasons to do so. When they express the conjugal act during infertile periods, they do not voluntarily will a child in that expression even though they are willing to accept a child lovingly if a conception were to occur. A separation of consequence occurs in that the conjugal act occurs without conception. The fact that particular expressions of the conjugal act do not result in procreation does not eliminate the divinely established connection between conjugal union and the conception of a child.

E. THE SACRIFICE OF PERIODIC ABSTINENCE

Since the conjugal act is important for marital harmony, Paul VI addresses near the beginning of *Humanae vitae*, the challenges of periodic abstinence: "Is not a reconsideration especially appropriate if it is believed that these norms cannot be observed without serious sacrifices [*gravia incommoda*], sometimes heroic sacrifices?"[65] Von Hildebrand formulates Paul VI's question as a claim: "It is frequently argued that abstaining from the conjugal act during the fertile days of the wife is too great a sacrifice."[66] If abstinence is not possible, then Paul VI's affirmation that the rhythm method is a moral means to postpone conception is simply a thought experiment. Spouses are left either with no means for postponing children or with use of artificial birth control.

Von Hildebrand argues with Paul VI that the abstinence required by the rhythm method is possible. He places the sacrifice of abstaining from the conjugal act within the context of God's general call for all Christians to take up their cross.[67] In requiring sacrifice, abstinence does not demand anything more than Christianity has always required. Christians are morally obliged to accept even death when it can be avoided only by sin. Von Hildebrand writes, "He who does not understand this is no Christian."[68]

Von Hildebrand contends that the sacrifice involved in temporary abstinence is often exaggerated: "How many people, for example, are ready to undertake temporary abstinence for professional reasons, such as prolonged journeys. I would not like to ask how many couples would be willing to abstain temporarily if they were offered a sum of money for every day of abstinence."[69] If spouses can abstain for business or financial reasons, then certainly they can abstain for the good of their family.

Von Hildebrand also responds to the position that "the calculation of days destroys spontaneity of the conjugal act and harms love."[70] The claim is true insofar as spontaneity is understood as mere impulse or instinct.[71] However, "it would be a symptom of a poor love and a weak sensuality, if the avoidance of all preliminary practical consideration, were necessary for spontaneity."[72] While von Hildebrand affirms the general relevance of spontaneity in expressing the conjugal act, he insists that since the conjugal act is a spiritual action, the handing over of one's self to mere instinct is what harms love not temporary abstinence.[73]

In marriage, spouses commit themselves to making sacrifices for the well-being of their beloved. Temporary abstinence, for spouses who mutually accept the sacrifice, may lead to "a special actualization of their love."[74] Insofar as spouses have discerned that the best thing for their family is to postpone having children, temporary abstinence is an expression of love. In fact, temporary abstinence can purify spouses' intentions for expressing the conjugal act. By discerning when to express and when to abstain from the conjugal act, spouses understand the action in relation to their marriage and to their conjugal love. Therefore, the sacrifice of temporary abstinence helps married couples "avoid the danger of treating the conjugal act merely as a means of sexual satisfaction."[75]

Abstaining from the conjugal act does not entail eliminating all expressions of conjugal love. Von Hildebrand writes, "The union desired in wedded love can and should find many expressions—from holding each other's hand, to the kiss on the lips, and the tender embrace."[76] While the conjugal act "represents the climax of this union," von Hildebrand maintains that "it is indeed deplorable when mutual wedded love is not expressed in many noble and tender displays of affection, when the manifestation of wedded love and of longing for union is restricted to the conjugal act."[77] Temporary abstinence, when placed within the context of marriage and the well-being of one's spouse and one's family, does not destroy conjugal love or the authenticity of the conjugal act but provides a unique actualization of conjugal love and purifies spouses' motives for expressing the conjugal act.

Von Hildebrand maintains the possibility of abstinence even when the situation requires that spouses postpone conception permanently. In particular, he notes the unique sacrifice of spouses who, because they are unable to determine their fertility, must commit themselves to life-long abstinence.[78] To resolve such situations, von Hildebrand joins Pius XII and Paul VI in expressing hope and prayer that "science will soon provide us with a means for detecting the days of fecundity in such a strict manner that the use of rhythm will become a reliable way of avoiding conception."[79] In the meantime, however, while von Hildebrand acknowledges the challenges of permanent abstinence, he concludes, "Though a great sacrifice be demanded of those married couples who cannot determine the fecund days with certainty, we nevertheless know that *no sacrifice* will detain the true Christian from obeying God's holy law. . . . Every true Christian is conscious of the deep and rudimentary meaning of sacrifice in this earthly life."[80]

F. SUMMARY

In his response to the 1930 Lambeth Conference, von Hildebrand argues that while recourse to the rhythm method is a morally acceptable means to prevent procreation, artificial birth control is not. At the time, his affirmation about the rhythm method was perhaps the more contentious stance in the Church. The general use of the rhythm method as a means to preventing conception does not receive Roman approval until Pius XII's 1951 address to the Italian Catholic Society of Midwives. Nonetheless, von Hildebrand speaks confidently on the issue, drawing from the framework he established in his works on *Purity* and *Marriage*. He maintains that the conjugal act has meaning in addition to procreation, namely, as the consummation of marriage and the actualization of conjugal love. Therefore, if spouses have significant reasons to postpone procreation, they may avoid procreation by only expressing the conjugal act in periods of perceived infertility. In using the rhythm method, spouses do not act immorally since the conjugal act is a spiritual act to be expressed freely and since God has established the conjugal act such that procreation does not always result.

Von Hildebrand indirectly affirms spouses' general responsibility to procreate and educate children when he affirms that spouses should prevent conception only when they have serious reasons for doing so. While von Hildebrand says little about the God-given mission of parents to procreate and educate children, his account both implicitly affirms this mission and provides a rich framework within which such discussion can flourish.

Von Hildebrand focuses his analysis on questions about nature and the possibility of periodic abstinence. Concerning the question of nature, he distinguishes between two understandings of the term. He remarks that "nature" can refer to the purely factual order of things or deeply meaningful relations. The former can be manipulated when necessary while the latter should not be changed. Recourse of the rhythm method to prevent conception is morally acceptable because it does not violate the deeply meaningful, divinely established connection between the conjugal act and procreation. Spouses who use the rhythm method to postpone pregnancy do not alter God's created order but respect the nature of that order.

Periodic abstinence is morally acceptable and concretely possible. Von Hildebrand emphasizes that to be a Christian means to accept and to endure suffering. Abstinence need not detract from conjugal love. If the spouses have responsibly discerned the need to postpone having children, their abstinence can be an expression of love and concern. By abstaining for a time spouses are less likely to be selfish in their expression of the conjugal act and more likely to understand the conjugal act as an actualization of love. For those spouses who have to endure permanent abstinence, von Hildebrand acknowledges their unique sacrifice. As a response to such situations, von Hildebrand encourages better understanding both of the meaning of suffering and the divinely established link between the conjugal act and procreation.

Notes

1. I am employing the term rhythm method because that was the term used and understanding of natural fertility available to von Hildebrand. Knowledge of a woman's cycle has significantly improved since von Hildebrand's works. Spouses now can more accurately identify when procreation might result through the monitoring of temperature, mucus, and the woman's cervix. These various ways of understanding a woman's cycle with the intention of having children or postponing pregnancy are categorized as methods of natural family planning. The rhythm method refers to the monitoring of a woman's fertility through attentiveness to the length of her periods. If a woman's period cycle was consistent then spouses could pinpoint when they are more likely to conceive a child. If spouses wanted to postpone having children they would reserve expression of the conjugal act for later in the woman's cycle. The rhythm method was developed by Kyusaku Ogino and Hermann Knaus in the 1920s and 1930s and popularized by Leo Latz. When von Hildebrand writes his article, "Lambeth-Botschaft," he does not indicate knowledge of Ogino and Knaus' research. The effectiveness of the methods available do not change his moral evaluation of whether or not spouses may prevent pregnancy through attentiveness to the woman's cycle and abstinence during those time periods when

pregnancy is most likely to occur. For more information on where Ogino and Knaus's research historically fits with debates in the Catholic tradition concerning the moral permissibility of the rhythm method, see John Noonan Jr., *Contraception: A History of Its Treatment by the Catholic Theologians and Canonists*, enlarged ed. (Cambridge, MA: Harvard University Press, 1986), 442-47 and William H. Shannon, *The Lively Debate: Response to Humanae Vitae* (New York: Sheed and Ward, 1970), 24-31.

2. *Man and Woman*, 102; note the similarity between von Hildebrand's discussion of changing notions of procreation and that of Augustine (Augustine, *On the Good of Marriage*, trans. C. L. Cornish, 403, in *Nicene and Post Nicene Fathers*, vol. 3, ed. Philip Schaff [Peabody, MA: Hendrickson Publishers, 1994]; see also 407). Note also that overpopulation was a stated concern in *Gaudium et spes* and *Humanae vitae* (Vatican II, *Gaudium et spes*, trans. Ronan Lennon, in *Vatican Council II: The Conciliar and Post Conciliar Documents*, new rev. ed., ed. Austin Flannery [Collegeville, MN: Liturgical Press, 1975], section 47, paragraph 2; see *AAS* 58 [1966]: 1067; Paul VI, *Humanae vitae*, trans. Janet Smith, in *Humanae Vitae: A Generation Later* [Washington, D.C.: The Catholic University of America, 1991], section 2, paragraph 1, 273, brackets in work cited; see also section 23, 289-90; *AAS* 60 [1968]: 481-82 and 497-98). I choose to use Smith's translation for a number of reasons. Smith states that while the encyclical originally was composed in Italian and French, she has translated the text from the Latin. She explains that "Latin remains the official language of the Church and thus the Latin version of *Humanae vitae* is the official text." She also affirms that "the Latin has important correspondences with earlier Church writings and serves better to show the continuity and development of certain arguments" (Smith, 269-70). Further, Smith explains that her translation was done in consultation with the original Italian. In addition to the reasons Smith provides for use of her translation, I employ Smith's translation because she is particularly astute and attentive to details concerning procreation's role in marriage.

3. *Man and Woman*, 100; John Paul II, in his apostolic exhortation *Familiaris consortio*, takes a more critical stance toward the issue of overpopulation. On one hand, he "recognizes the serious problem of population growth in the form it has taken in many parts of the world and its moral implications" (John Paul II, *Familiaris consortio* trans. anonymous (Vatican: Vatican Polyglot Press, 1981, section 31, paragraph 1, 58; *AAS* 74 [1982]: 117). On the other hand, he speaks of a growing "anti-life mentality" which is evidenced among other things by "a certain panic deriving from the studies of ecologists and futurologists on population growth, which sometimes exaggerate the danger of demographic increase to the quality of life" (*Familiaris consortio*, section 30, paragraph 3, 56). In the *AAS* version, the phrase "anti-life mentality" is stated in Latin and then listed with italics in parenthesis in English (*AAS* 74 [1982]: 116). See also Carl Olson's review of *Man and Woman*, where Olson criticizes von Hildebrand's work on the issue of overpopulation (Carl Olson, review of *Man, Woman, and the Meaning of Love*, by Dietrich von Hildebrand, *National Catholic Register* 78, 34 [Aug 25-31 2002]: 14). For his part, von Hildebrand questions why those concerned about overpopulation are not speaking against artificial insemination (*Man and Woman*, 100). For a more thorough critique of overpopulation theories see Jacqueline Kasun, *The War Against Population: The Economics and Ideology of World Population Control* (San Francisco, CA: Ignatius Press, 1988) and Mercedes Arzú Wilson, *Love and Family: Raising a Traditional Family in a Secular World* (San Francisco, CA: Ignatius Press, 1996).

4. *Man and Woman*, 102.

5. *Man and Woman*, 84.

6. *Man and Woman*, 103. The list of questions that precede this answer is as follows: "Could anyone claim that this new situation also affects the vocation of marriage, that fewer people should get married, or that a man and a woman, loving each other with spousal love, should renounce the union of marriage for the sake of avoiding the increase of population? Or could one even claim that bodily union loses, by that, its justification, and that one should encourage married people to live in abstinence, though they feel not the slightest vocation for a virginal marriage? Or may one argue that man's intervention by artificial birth control is warranted by circumstances even though it is a sin?" (*Man and Woman*, 102-103).

7. "Lambeth-Botschaft," 27, my translation. The original reads as follows: "Ja, die hl. Poenitentiarie erklärte sogar, daß es Eheleuten, die aus sittlich berechtigten Gründen Nachkom-

menschaft zeitweilig vermeiden wollen, erlaubt sei, Tage mit fakultativer Sterilität auszuwählen für die geschlechtliche Vereinigung."

8. "Onanism" is when a man, during sexual intercourse, intentionally ejaculates outside of the participating woman's vagina. The term points back to the actions of Onan in Genesis chapter 38: "Onan, however, knew that the descendants would not be counted as his; so whenever he had relations with his brother's widow, he wasted his seed on the ground" (Gen. 38:9, *New American Bible*). See also Noonan's description of how "onanism" was understood in the late nineteenth century (Noonan, 397-98).

9. Noonan, 441.

10. Noonan, 443; Pius XI did not address directly the question of the rhythm method in his encyclical *Casti connubii*. He does affirm, however, that offspring could be avoided through "virtuous continence (which Christian law permits in matrimony when both parties consent" (Pius XI, *On Christian Marriage*, trans. anonymous [Boston, MA: St. Paul Editions, neither the publication date nor the translation are listed; the cover states, "Official Vatican Text"], paragraph 54, 92; *AAS* 22 [1930]: 559). Pius XI also writes, "Nor are those considered as acting against nature who in the married state use their right in the proper manner although on account of natural reasons either of time or of certain defects, new life cannot be brought forth" (Pius XI, paragraph 59, 30).

11. Noonan, 446; Pius XII states, "If the carrying out of this theory means nothing more than that the couple can make use of their matrimonial rights on the days of natural sterility too, there is nothing against it, for by so doing they neither hinder nor injure in any way the consummation of the natural act and its further natural consequences" (Pius XII, "The Apostolate of the Midwife," in *The Major Addresses of Pope Pius XII*, vol. 1, ed. Vincent A. Yzermans [St. Paul, MN: North Central Publishing, 1961], 168; *AAS* 43 [1951]: 844).

12. Noonan paraphrases John Ryan's stance on how the 1880 statement could be interpreted: "the 1880 answer of the Penitentiary could be liberally construed to permit confessors to suggest the sterile period not only to those already practicing contraception, but to any married person with a serious reason for avoiding offspring" (Noonan, 443; Noonan is paraphrasing John A. Ryan, "The Moral Aspects of Periodical Continence,"*Ecclesiastical Review* 89 (1933): 29 and 37-38). Noonan does not provide proper pagination for Ryan's article. He indicates that Ryan discusses the matter on page 28 of his article but Ryan does not discuss the 1880 Penitentiary statement until page 29 and then again at 37-38. Ryan argues that the 1880 statement should not be read strictly as if to say that confessors can recommend recourse to infertile periods only to prevent "onanism" and in no other situation. Ryan argues that the 1880 statement leaves open the possibility for confessors to recommend use of infertile periods to prevent use of contraception. He argues this for three reasons: 1) the statement was addressing the question of "onanism" and had no reason to speak to the issue of contraception; 2) knowledge of the infertile period was limited (actually misleading) in 1880; 3) knowledge of preventing conception through contraceptives or restrictive intercourse was less general in 1880 (Ryan, 37). Nonetheless, Ryan highlights that the 1880 statement indicates that confessors must exercise "prudence and discretion" in recommending recourse to the infertile periods (Ryan, 38).

13. On the issue of whether the conjugal act has meaning in addition to procreation, see also *Gaudium et spes*, which states, "marriage is not merely for the procreation of children: its nature as an indissoluble compact between two people and the good of children demand that the mutual love of the partners be properly shown, that it should grow and mature. Even in cases where despite the intense desire of the spouses there are no children, marriage still retains its character of being a whole manner and communion of life and preserves its value and indissolubility" (section 50, paragraph 3, 954); see also *Humanae vitae*, where Paul VI writes, "Conjugal acts do not cease being legitimate if the spouses are aware that they are infertile for reasons not voluntarily caused by them; these acts remain ordained [*destinatio*] to expressing and strengthening the union of the spouses" (section 11, paragraph 1, 280, brackets in work cited).

14. *The Encyclical "Humanae Vitae,"* 47, italics in work cited.

15. He writes in "Lambeth-Botschaft," that "to practice abstinence except on certain days with the wish to avoid children out of serious grounds, perhaps portrays a certain becoming independent of the meaning of the marital union and an elimination of the end . . ." (Lambeth-Botschaft, 27, my translation). The German reads as follows: "Enthaltsamkeit üben, außer an

gewissen Tagen, mit dem Wunsch, aus schwerwiegenden Gründen sich Kinder versagen zu müssen, stellt wohl eine gewisse Verselbständigung des Sinnes der ehelichen Vereinigung und eine Ausschaltung des Zweckes derselben dar . . ."

16. See "Lambeth-Botschaft," 27, where von Hildebrand writes, "It certainly is necessary that the conjugal act be seen in the light of conceiving a child" (my translation; the German reads: "Es ist wohl erforderlich, daß er generell im Licht der Zeugung eines neuen Menschen gesehen wird"); see also *Marriage*, 23.

17. "Lambeth-Botschaft," 27, my translation. The original German for these two phrases is respectively, "aus sittlich berechtigten Gründen" and "aus schwerwiegenden Gründen."

18. *The Encyclical "Humanae Vitae,"* 37 and 47; the original German is respectively "aus legitmen Gründen" and "aus ernsten Gründen" (*Die Enzyklika*, 24 and 30).

19. *The Nature of Love*, 156.

20. *The Nature of Love*, 197-98.

21. *The Nature of Love*, 197 and 368-69.

22. *The Nature of Love*, 197 and 367-68.

23. Pius XII, 173-74, I have included the content in parentheses which comes from the original Italian provided in *AAS* 43 (1951): 850-51; see also Janet Smith's discussion of the "extreme value given to procreation" in Scripture (Smith, 129-33).

24. *Gaudium et spes*, section 48, paragraph 2, 951. Immediately following this quote, the Council Fathers emphasize the unique sacramental graces of marriage which fortify and consecrate "the duty and dignity of their state."

25. *Gaudium et spes*, section 50, paragraph 1, 953; see also section 50, paragraph 2, 953.

26. Smith, 136, quoting *Humanae vitae*, section one, paragraph one, Smith adds the content in parentheses.

27. Smith, 136, quoting *Gaudium et spes*, section 51, paragraph 4, 955 as found in *Vatican Council II: The Conciliar and Post Conciliar Documents*. Smith adds the content in parentheses since the term *munus* is dropped in the translation. This quote concludes the second to last section in the marriage segment of *Gaudium et spes*. Smith argues that the two phrases should be read together because of the common use of *munus* and because the one quote is placed near the end of *Gaudium et spes* and the other at the beginning of *Humanae vitae*. In addition, the two documents are connected because certain questions raised during the formation of *Gaudium et spes* were postponed for further consideration. In a footnote just prior to the noted use of *munus*, the Council Fathers write, "By order of the Holy Father, certain questions requiring further and more careful investigation have been given over to a commission for the study of population, the family, and births, in order that the Holy Father may pass judgment when its task is completed. With the teaching of the magisterium standing as it is, the Council has no intention of proposing concrete solutions at this moment" (*Gaudium et spes*, footnote to section 51, paragraph 3, 955).

28. Smith, 137; Smith also writes that the word *munus* gives one "access to a dimension of the encyclical often neglected, a dimension that stresses the positive aspect of having children" (p. 136).

29. Smith, 140.

30. Smith, 137.

31. *Humanae vitae*, section one, paragraph 1, 272, brackets in work cited.

32. *Familiaris consortio*, section 28, paragraph 1, 53; see also section 28, paragraph 2, 53.

33. *Gaudium et spes*, section 48, paragraph 1 and section 50, paragraph 1, 950 and 953; Paul VI repeats the latter quote in *Humanae vitae*, section 9, paragraph 5, 279, a quote that is then repeated by John Paul II in *Familiaris consortio*, 14, 1, 26.

34. *Familiaris consortio*, section 30, paragraph 4, 56; since children are a gift, spouses should not view them as a burden but welcome them with joy. Pius XII encourages midwives to "instill in the mind and heart of the mother and the father esteem, desire, and joy for the newborn child" (Pius XII, 163). Similarly, John Paul II writes, "I repeat once again what I said to the General Assembly of the United Nations on October 2, 1979: 'I wish to express the joy that we all find in children, the springtime of life, the anticipation of the future history of each of our present earthly homelands'" (*Familiaris consortio*, section 26, paragraph 3, 50).

35. *Familiaris consortio*, section 38, paragraph 3, 75; see also section 15, paragraph 2, 28; section 21, paragraph 5, 41; and section 39, paragraph 2, 76-77; and *Gaudium et spes*, section 48, paragraph 3, 951.

36. *Gaudium et spes*, section 50, paragraph 1, 953; see also section 48, paragraph 4, 951-52.

37. *Familiaris consortio*, section 21, paragraph 6, 41.

38. Smith, 145.

39. *Gaudium et spes*, section 52, paragraph 2, 956; see also *Familiaris consortio*, section 46, paragraph 3, 87.

40. Pius XI, paragraph 120, 64.

41. *Familiaris consortio*, section 30, paragraph 6, 57; see also von Hildebrand's remarks on this issue in *Man and Woman*: "The question of how many children a couple has is, as such, patently not within the realm of competence of the state. The state has not the right to forbid a marriage in which children cannot be expected, nor to set a *numerus clauses* for children" (p. 101).

42. *Humanae vitae*, section 10, paragraph 1, 279.

43. *Humanae vitae*, section 10, paragraph 5, 280, brackets in work cited.

44. *Humanae vitae*, section 10, paragraph 6, 280.

45. Pius XII, 168; he also writes that if "there are no similar grave reasons of a personal nature or deriving from external circumstances, then the determination to avoid habitually the fecundity of the union while at the same time to continue satisfying their sensuality, can be derived only from a false appreciation of life and from reasons having nothing to do with proper ethical laws" (Pius XII, 169).

46. *Gaudium et spes*, section 51, paragraph 1, 954.

47. *Humanae vitae*, section 10, paragraph 4, 279-80.

48. Pius XII, 169.

49. *Humanae vitae*, section 10, paragraph 4, 279; see also, section 16, paragraph 2, 284-85.

50. *Gaudium et spes*, section 50, paragraph 2, 954.

51. *Humanae vitae*, section 10, paragraph 4, 279.

52. For further discussion on responsible parenthood, see Janet E. Smith, "The Moral Use of Natural Family Planning," in *Why Humanae Vitae Was Right: A Reader*, ed. Janet E. Smith (San Francisco, CA: Ignatius Press, 1993), 445-71.

53. Paul VI, *Humanae vitae*, section 16, paragraph 3, 285, brackets in work cited. Paul VI repeats the importance of nature throughout his work often with reference to earlier works; see *Humanae vitae*, section 9, paragraph 4, 279 and section 10, paragraph 6, 280, where Paul VI quotes and paraphrases remarks from *Gaudium et spes*, see *Gaudium et spes*, sections 50-51, 953-55; see also *Humanae vitae*, section 11, paragraph 1, 281, where Paul VI paraphrases both Pius XI's *Casti connubii* and Pius XII, who also quotes Pius XI in his address, "The Apostolate of the Midwife" (see *Casti connubii*, paragraph 56, 29 and Pius XII, 167).

54. Paul VI notes the general importance of nature when posing the initial questions of the encyclical. He writes, "Finally, and above all, it must be noted that because Man has made such remarkable progress in controlling [*moderandis*] the forces of nature and in rationally organizing them, he also strives to extend this control [*moderationem*] to the whole of his life: that is, to his body, to the powers of his mind [*ad sui animi vires*], to his social life, and even to the laws that regulate the propagation of life" (*Humanae vitae*, section 2, paragraph 3, 273, brackets in work cited).

55. *The Encyclical "Humanae Vitae,"* 39; see also 40.

56. Other examples that von Hildebrand provides of purely factual relationships include the proximity of the esophagus to the windpipe, the removal of a cancerous uterus, and a heart transplant (*The Encyclical "Humanae Vitae,"* 39-41). When Paul VI addresses the question of how man may legitimately intervene to "restrain the irrational forces of nature" he affirms that use of the human intellect "must be done in accord with the order or reality [*rerum ordine*] established by God" (*Humanae vitae*, section 16, paragraph 1, brackets in work cited).

57. *The Encyclical "Humanae Vitae,"* 39.

58. *The Encyclical "Humanae Vitae,"* 40, italics in work cited.

59. *The Encyclical "Humanae Vitae,"* 39-40.

60. See Janet Smith's analysis of different natural law arguments in relation to *Humanae vitae* in her work *Humanae Vitae: A Generation Later*, 68-128 and 161-229.

61. *The Encyclical "Humanae Vitae,"* 40.

62. *The Encyclical "Humanae Vitae,"* 40.

63. *The Encyclical "Humanae Vitae,"* 47; see also 38.

64. "Lambeth-Botschaft," 28, my translation; the German reads as follows: "Die Wahl des Augenblickes, wann dieses Land betreten wird, steht dem Menschen in der Ehe frei." See also "Lambeth-Botschaft," 27. Pius XII makes a similar remark in his address to midwives: "Nature puts at man's disposal the whole chain of causes giving rise to a new human life: it is man who has to release the living force, nature that must develop its course and bring it to completion. Once man has performed his part and put into motion this wondrous evolution of life, his duty forbids his arresting the work of nature or hindering its natural development" (Pius XII, 161).

65. *Humanae vitae*, section 3, paragraph 1, 273-74.

66. *The Encyclical "Humanae Vitae,"* 53; Paul VI writes, "The teaching of the Church about the proper spacing of children is a promulgation of the divine law itself. No doubt many will think this teaching difficult, if not impossible, to keep" (*Humanae vitae*, section 20, 288).

67. *The Encyclical "Humanae Vitae,"* 53; see also John Paul II, *Familiaris consortio*, section 34, paragraph 5, 67-68.

68. *The Encyclical "Humanae Vitae,"* 53.

69. *The Encyclical "Humanae Vitae,"* 54.

70. *The Encyclical "Humanae Vitae,"* 53.

71. *The Encyclical "Humanae Vitae,"* 54.

72. *The Encyclical "Humanae Vitae,"* 55.

73. *The Encyclical "Humanae Vitae,"* 54-55; see also Pius XII, 173-74 and *Humanae vitae*, section 21, 288-89.

74. *The Encyclical "Humanae Vitae,"* 54; see also Paul VI, *Humanae vitae*, section 21, paragraphs 1-2, 288-89; Paul VI's remarks are repeated by John Paul II in *Familiaris consortio*, section 33, paragraph 8, 65-66.

75. *The Encyclical "Humanae Vitae,"* 54.

76. *The Encyclical "Humanae Vitae,"* 55.

77. *The Encyclical "Humanae Vitae,"* 55-56.

78. *The Encyclical "Humanae Vitae,"* 54 and 61.

79. *Man and Woman*, 100; see also 102; von Hildebrand notes Pius XII's request for prayer in both *Man and Woman*, 100 and *The Encyclical "Humanae Vitae,"* 48. In the latter work, he also notes that Paul VI repeats Pius XII's request in *Humanae vitae*, section 24, 290-91; see also *Gaudium et spes*, section 52, paragraph 4, 957. Thirteen years after *Humanae vitae*, John Paul II writes, "The Church notes with satisfaction the results achieved by scientific research aimed at a more precise knowledge of the rhythms of women's fertility" (*Familiaris consortio*, section 35, paragraph 2, 69). He then expresses the need for those who know about human fertility to effectively teach others. He writes that the Church "cannot fail to call with renewed vigor on the responsibility of all—doctors, experts, marriage counselors, teachers and married couples—who can actually help married people to live their love with respect for the structure and finalities of the conjugal act which expresses that love. This implies a broader, more decisive and more systematic effort to make the natural methods of regulating fertility known, respected and applied" (*Familiaris consortio*, section 35, paragraph 2, 69; see also section 33, paragraph 7, 64-65).

80. *The Encyclical "Humanae Vitae,"* 61, italics in work cited; see also Pius XII's statement concerning the requirement of complete abstinence: "God does not oblige people to do the impossible. But God obliges married people to abstain, if their union cannot be fulfilled according to the laws of nature. Therefore, in this case abstinence is possible" (Pius XII, 170).

Chapter Six

Artificial Birth Control

Von Hildebrand's academic career encompasses two of the most consequential documents concerning artificial birth control, the 1930 Anglican Conference at Lambeth and Paul VI's 1968 encyclical, *Humanae vitae*. The context in which the Anglican leaders and Paul VI issued their statements stands in such contrast that one easily forgets that only thirty-eight years separate the documents. The Anglican leaders' sanction of spousal use of artificial birth control was the first time in Christian history that Christian leaders had formally approved of the practice.[1] The surprise of *Humanae vitae* was not a change in the tradition but the fact that Paul VI did not change the Church's stance despite significant speculation that he would do so. Amid the changing currents of the mid-twentieth century, von Hildebrand offers a remarkable consistency of thought. His analysis of artificial birth control focuses on three themes: conjugal love, reverence, and conscience.

A. CONJUGAL LOVE AND ARTIFICIAL BIRTH CONTROL

Von Hildebrand's "Lambeth-Botschaft" and *The Encyclical "Humanae Vitae"* work within the framework of conjugal love. In his response to the Lambeth Conference, he commends the document's analysis of conjugal love but argues that the document fails on the important issue of birth control. He maintains that insights into conjugal love do not imply the moral acceptability of artificial birth control.[2] His defense of *Humanae vitae* is in part a defense of his own thought. In his earlier works, he had proposed that conjugal love was the primary meaning of marriage and in the 1960s theologians were using similar positions to justify artificial birth control. Paul VI testifies to this development in reasoning when he writes, "many who attempt to defend artificial ways of limiting the number of children give as their reason the demands of conjugal love."[3] If the conjugal act has meaning as an actualization of conjugal love even when conception does not occur, then what is wrong with preventing procreation through contraception?

Von Hildebrand was not oblivious to possible misunderstandings of his earlier proposal. In *Purity*, after asserting that spouses, in expressing the conjugal act, should seek not only the end of procreation but also "the expression and fulfillment of wedded love," he clarifies in a footnote: "The fact that the act of marriage also possesses a significance for man, *in quantum homo*—namely, the expression and fulfillment of wedded love—is of course no justification whatsoever for an artificial divorce of this purpose from the function of generation."[4] To affirm that marriage and the conjugal act have goods in addition to procreation is not to deny procreation's central role.

Von Hildebrand repeats his criticism of artificial birth control in *Marriage*, "Lambeth-Botschaft," *Art of Living*, and *Man and Woman*. And yet, he does not seem able to escape the further question, even though he himself does not support contraception, does his account of marriage and the conjugal act lean in that direction? Von Hildebrand addresses this question in the introduction to his work, *The Encyclical "Humanae Vitae"*:

> For years, I have defended the position that marriage, as well as the marital act, has meaning not only because of procreation, but also as the expression and fulfillment of a deep union of love. It was occasionally said that by affirming that the marital act retains a meaning and high value even when—through no intervention of ours—conception cannot occur, I was opening the door to a justification of artificial birth control. But this approach showed a misapprehension of my position, for I had emphatically stated in many articles and books that artificial birth control cannot be allowed. It was precisely my intention to call attention to the great mystery of God's having entrusted the generation of a new human being to the most intimate union of love. The dignity and beauty of the marital act as an irrevocable mutual self-donation in which the two spouses become "one flesh" cause the mysterious link between this act and the birth of a new human being to shine forth in all nobility and grandeur.[5]

He argues that if one understands his account of conjugal love, then one will see with greater detail why artificial birth control is a sin: "the question of birth control must be considered in the light of the mystery of true love and its fulfillment in bodily donation and never in terms of sexual attraction—today so often called 'love.'"[6] To advocate use of artificial birth control on the basis of conjugal love is to misunderstand conjugal love.

The conjugal act is both an actualization of conjugal love and ordered to procreation: "both constituents have been so organically united by God that to disrupt this unity by breaking this mysterious and solemn bond between the different factors must be on that account, if for no other reason, a frightful sacrilege."[7] On the one hand, spouses' failure to actualize conjugal love in the marital act "is the source of all *impurity*."[8] On the other hand, "the *active*, artificial isolation of this act from the possible generation of a human being constitutes a sin of *irreverence* toward God. This is usurping a right not given to the creature."[9] For von Hildebrand, if one is able to see the divinely established connection between conjugal love and the conjugal act, then one is more likely to see the divinely ordained link between procreation and the conjugal act, and vice versa.

B. REVERENCE AND ARTIFICIAL BIRTH CONTROL

Von Hildebrand describes contraceptive acts in contrast to spousal prevention of conception through use of the rhythm method.[10] He acknowledges that in both cases, spouses express sexual union without the intention of offspring.[11] He approaches the distinction by asking a series of questions:

> Why shouldn't man be allowed to regulate birth by artificial means, when God, after all, gave man control and dominion over nature and in the Old Testament made him the master of creation? Why is it allowed in medicine to take out the uterus, to transplant hearts, and perform many kinds of operations, but forbidden to intervene and modify nature in the case of the regulation of births?[12]

He responds in part by explaining the meaning of man's dominion over creation. Dominion over nature does not entail that one can do whatever he wants to nature but recognition that God "entrusts to man's free will the task of harmonizing things as they are with things as they ought to be."[13]

God addresses man's freedom when He gives him dominion over creation. One *should* respect and cultivate the order of creation. Accordingly, the divinely established connection between the conjugal act and procreation is "a profoundly mysterious area of creation, where what is can either coincide with what ought to be or deviate from it."[14] The faculty of human freedom enables man to "do what he *ought not* do . . . a causal sequence is not deprived of its efficacy because men abuse it."[15]

God, who alone is Creator, has greatly honored spouses by allowing them to participate in something only He can do, namely, create new life. Since this domain belongs uniquely to God, spouses should respect the means by which God allows them to participate in His work.

Von Hildebrand is concerned not only with the general fact that the conjugal act leads to procreation, but with identifying the particular way that God links the conjugal act with procreation. He notes that procreation does not result from every expression of the conjugal act. The conjugal act should be an actualization of conjugal love committed in marriage from which procreation flows as a superabundant fruit. That procreation does not always result from the conjugal act is, for von Hildebrand, a word from God highlighting the mystery that creation flows from an act of love and that the conjugal act retains meaning when procreation does not result. When spouses have serious need to postpone or prevent pregnancy, they may employ the rhythm method in which spouses seek to understand the God-established relationship between the conjugal act and procreation. They respect that relationship and leave the connection intact. Spouses who use artificial birth control to prevent pregnancy manipulate the divinely ordained link between procreation and the conjugal act. In so doing, they commit a grave sin of irreverence before their Creator.[16]

Von Hildebrand often repeats his claim that use of artificial birth control involves a sin of irreverence. In *Marriage*, he writes, "It is difficult to imagine a greater lack of reverence toward God than interfering with this mystery with desecrating hands."[17] In his "Lambeth-Botschaft" article, he describes contraception as "a presumptuous intervention in the mystery of human origins . . . a wicked intervention in a God-willed connection, even the violation of the mystery of this sphere"[18] and "a wicked, impudent violation of the mysterious character of this sphere, a presumptuous acting as Lord of this sphere, an irreverent change and reign which belongs especially to the reservation of God . . . an irreverent presumption against God."[19]

Von Hildebrand provides a perceptive summary of his argument against artificial birth control in his later work *Man and Woman*, a summary he then repeats in *The Encyclical "Humanae Vitae"*:

> The sinfulness of artificial birth control is rooted in the fact that one arrogates to oneself the right to separate the actualized love union in marriage from a possible procreation, to sever this wonderful, deeply mysterious connection, instituted by God, approaching this mystery in an irreverent attitude. We are here confronted with the basic sin or irreverence toward God, the denial of our creaturehood, the acting as if we were our own lords. It is the basic denial of the *religio*, of our being bound to God; it is a disrespect for the mysteries of God's creation, which increases in its sinfulness the higher the rank of the mystery in question. It is the same sinfulness which lies in suicide, or in euthanasia, in both of which we act as if we were masters of life.[20]

The sin of irreverence involved in use of artificial birth control is not a failure to engage in shallow piety but rather a failure to recognize one's basic place before God, that is, that one is a creature before the Creator.

The key issue for von Hildebrand in distinguishing between the rhythm method and artificial birth control is whether or not the spouses actively intervene and manipulate the means by which God has established for them to participate in His creative power. While one could say that spouses who intend to prevent pregnancy without serious reasons for doing so commit a sin of selfishness or at least show a lack of generosity, von Hildebrand argues that manipulating the means of creation involves the more fundamental sin of irreverence. Use of artificial birth control renders infertile sexual unions that would lead to the creation of new human life. Contraception "cuts off the creative intervention of God."[21]

The distinction between active intervention and letting the God-established connection unfold, for von Hildebrand, has application in those situations when one spouse employs artificial birth control against the will of the other spouse. Von Hildebrand maintains, "though no Catholic spouse is allowed to use contraceptive means, he is still not allowed to refuse the marital act even when his partner employs contraceptive means. Here also the distinction between the active and passive attitude is morally decisive."[22] The participating spouse, while opposed to his beloved using contraception, is himself not actively intervening against God's ordained link between the conjugal act and procreation, and is therefore free to grant the marriage right.[23]

Von Hildebrand insists that when conjugal love and the end of procreation are properly understood, spouses cannot pit the two against each other:

> It is a fiction to say that a couple wanting to follow the command of the Church but still conscious of their duty to preserve the stability and harmony of their marriage are forced to choose between two duties. Couples who are faithful children of the Church and eager to fulfill God's will could never consider the possibility of adultery as inevitable if they had to make the sacrifice of using rhythm in their marital life.[24]

To argue that one will commit a sin of impurity if not allowed to commit the sin of irreverence is an attempt to blackmail God.[25] The avoidance of one sin does not cause another sin. To give someone a choice between two sins is to lead him astray.

In his response to the 1930 Lambeth Conference, von Hildebrand argues that artificial birth control does not promote but hinders conjugal love. He proposes that contraception is "incompatible with a basic assumption of purity, which involves an awe before the mystery, a consciousness of being able to actualize the sexual sphere only with the express sanction of God, a reverent listening to and hearing of God's will."[26] Purity requires a disposition of reverence. Couples should understand conjugal love in light of Christ and they should both enter marriage and express the conjugal act only with God's sanction. For that reason, use of artificial birth control to prevent conception, and the irreverence it implies, undermines the possibility of purity and thereby undermines the development of conjugal love.

While von Hildebrand does not describe other negative consequences of artificial birth control, his discussion of reverence indicates that the effects of contraception on the moral life are disastrous. Reverence is the foundation for right relationship with God and therefore the foundation of the moral life. Reverence is required to respond to the goods of God's created order and for the development of all virtues. Once one has overthrown the Creator the moral life is open for revolution.

Von Hildebrand's discussion of reverence and identification of contraception as irreverent supports Paul VI and John Paul II's claims about the immorality that flows from use of artificial birth control. Paul VI predicts that use of contraception will lead many "to justify behavior leading to marital infidelity."[27] If one does not have reverence for God, then one will lack reverence for the commitment entailed in the sacrament of marriage. Further, one is more likely to express sexual union with someone other than one's spouse if one is tempted by the idea that a possible conception is stripped from such a union.

Paul VI also warns against "a gradual weakening in the discipline of morals."[28] He continues,

> Not much experience is needed to understand human weakness and to comprehend that human beings, especially the young, are so susceptible to temptation that they need to be encouraged to keep the moral law. It is wrong to make it easy for them to violate this law. Indeed, it is to be feared that husbands who become accustomed to contraceptive practices will lose respect for their wives. They may come to disregard their wife's psychological and physical equilibrium and use their wives as instruments for serving their own desires. Consequently, they will no longer view their wives as companions who should be treated with attentiveness and love.[29]

In other words, the same reasons that would tempt one to marital infidelity would tempt spouses to reduce the conjugal act from a spiritual, deep, and meaningful gift of self to a shallow, self-seeking, handing over of one's self to sexual pleasure. Spouses would be tempted to use their beloved merely for the sake of sexual gratification.

Thirdly, Paul VI warns that moral sanction of artificial birth control would lead public authorities to mandate contraception for their citizens:

> Would anyone blame those in the highest offices of the state for employing a solution [contraception] considered morally permissible for spouses seeking to solve a family difficulty, when they strive to solve certain difficulties affecting the whole nation? Who will prevent public authorities from favoring what they believe to be the most effective contraceptive methods and from mandating that everyone must use them, whenever they consider it necessary? And clearly it will come about that Men who desire to avoid the difficulties that are part of the divine law, difficulties that individuals, families, or society may experience, will hand over to the will of the public authorities the power of interfering in the most exclusive and intimate mission [*munus*] of spouses.[30]

Paul VI sees this possibility as a unique likelihood amid concern about overpopulation.[31] If the general public recognizes contraception as a moral means to prevent pregnancy and the world is overpopulated, then government leaders might publicly finance or even mandate use of contraception.

John Paul II, thirteen years later, stresses the negative impact of artificial birth control to such an extent that he speaks of a "truly contraceptive mentality."[32] Unlike Paul VI, his voice is not one warning about the future but one concerned about active practices. He writes that "the Church condemns as a grave offense against human dignity and justice all those activities of governments or other public authorities which attempt to limit in any way the freedom of couples in deciding about children."[33] He further critiques the "contraceptive mentality" in light of a "consumer mentality." He explains that while many families go without the basic goods necessary to raise children, for other families, "excessive prosperity and the consumer mentality . . . deprive married couples of the generosity and courage needed for raising up new human life: thus life is often perceived not as a blessing, but as a danger from which to defend oneself."[34] Ultimately, he concludes that the "reason for these mentalities is the absence in people's hearts of God, whose love alone is stronger than all the world's fears and can conquer them."[35] The evils of contraception flow from a basic failure of reverence.

C. CONSCIENCE AND ARTIFICIAL BIRTH CONTROL

Even though von Hildebrand published *The Encyclical "Humanae Vitae"* only a few months after *Humanae vitae*, his work indicates some of the immediate disapproval that greeted the encyclical. In his introduction, von Hildebrand places those opposed to Paul VI's condemnation of artificial birth control into two categories. He speaks on one hand of those "faithful married Catholics who, though uninfected by the movement of secularization, are understandably very disappointed; for . . . many spiritual advisors and confessors had been telling them that the use of the pill is morally unobjectionable should serious reasons for prevention of pregnancy arise."[36] On the other hand, he speaks of those who are "motivated by a general amoralism and a resentful rebellion against the Church and her teaching authority."[37]

For the second group, the hardships that the rhythm method poses for spouses provide "a welcome occasion for undermining respect for the Holy Father as well as faith in the teaching authority of the Holy Church."[38] Von Hildebrand concerns himself in particular with the argument that spouses should come to their own conclusion about contraception based on their conscience. He argues that this claim fails to understand conscience's role in the moral life. He proposes that one comes to know what is good or evil either by "the faculty of value perception" or by "a moral authority."[39] Accordingly, he affirms that "conscience does not instruct us about whether something is morally good or evil; rather, this question must be answered *before* conscience can speak."[40] He concludes that conscience's "primary function is to warn us not to do certain things—it is mainly concerned with the *avoidance* of immoral actions or the condemnation of past actions—though it also urges us to do good when failure to do so would be a sin."[41]

One's value perception (or value blindness) and not one's conscience reaches the conclusion about whether or not use of artificial birth control is morally good. Therefore, "it is spurious to say that the question of whether or not a couple submits to the papal prohibition of artificial birth control should be decided by their conscience."[42] The real issue is value perception. If one does not think artificial birth control is wrong then one's conscience will not warn against it.[43]

Since one comes to know the good not only through value perception but also by moral authority, the formation of conscience involves consideration of authority. Moral authority is necessary because "man's ability to grasp moral values is weakened by many factors."[44] For example, one struggles to perceive clearly the values in a decision (like the decision between the rhythm method and artificial birth control) when one choice involves sacrifice and the other does not: "even a pagan of high moral standard would assume that some morally trustworthy person whose personal wishes are not involved would be able to advise him more objectively as to his real duty."[45]

Von Hildebrand specifically is concerned with the claim that those who are "competent on matters of marriage and sexual ethics" may disregard Paul VI's condemnation of artificial birth control in *Humanae vitae*. He responds that while individuals with moral integrity may have a relative moral authority, "in faith and morals there is for the Catholic just one absolutely competent authority—the Church."[46] He maintains that Paul VI's condemnation of artificial birth control carries particular weight because the declaration was "a long awaited and dramatically important pronouncement, in accordance with the unbroken traditional teaching of the Church."[47] He asserts that those who oppose Paul VI's condemnation are not only approving a grave sin of irreverence but also disavowing their belief in the teaching authority of the Church.

Von Hildebrand critiques the position that Paul VI's condemnation of artificial birth control involves a conflict of conscience for spouses. He affirms that a "conflict of conscience arises only when an evil is being imposed by an authority. No one would say my conscience would forbid temporary abstinence."[48] Even for those who think artificial birth control is morally acceptable, if they affirm the teaching authority of the Church, they can proceed in good conscience through use of the rhythm method or abstinence.

Von Hildebrand proposes that "conscience does not speak a no against church statements but remains silent as I give into wishes and desires."[49]

While recognizing the difficulties of those married couples who had previously been advised to use artificial birth control, von Hildebrand ultimately concludes that "no misfortune—however great—is commensurate with the fearful disharmony issuing from an offense of God. . . . sin has an eternal resonance, whereas all other evils are restricted to the temporal order. The pagan, Socrates, said: 'It is better for man to suffer injustice that to commit it'"[50] He had reached a similar conclusion nearly forty years earlier, when he wrote that "in the use of contraception lies a serious sin, which not even justified motives, such as consideration of health, or the economic impossibility or raising children can make permissible."[51]

D. SUMMARY

Von Hildebrand's academic career spanned the unique time frame enabling him to offer published responses to both the 1930 Lambeth Conference and Paul VI's 1968 encyclical, *Humanae vitae*. Although the context in which these two ecclesial documents were issued varied considerably, von Hildebrand's responses show remarkable consistency. Von Hildebrand's discussion of artificial birth control focuses on conjugal love, reverence, and conscience.

While von Hildebrand's *The Encyclical "Humanae Vitae"* is a defense of Paul VI, one should also see in this short work a defense of von Hildebrand's own thought. Earlier in his career, von Hildebrand had defended the claim that in addition to the primary end of procreation, marriage and the conjugal act also have the primary meaning of conjugal love. He was concerned in affirming the foundational role of conjugal love not to undermine the centrality of procreation. Accordingly, he argues in *Purity* and "Lambeth-Botschaft" that recognition of conjugal love's value does not entail support of artificial birth control. He writes in the introduction to *The Encyclical "Humanae Vitae"* that while some have proposed that his writings have opened the door for use of artificial birth control a proper understanding of conjugal love actually highlights the evil of contraception.

Von Hildebrand places conjugal love within the realm of one's relationship to God and thereby relates conjugal love to the virtue of reverence. In reverence, spouses recognize that God alone is Creator and that he greatly honors them in enabling them to participate in His creative action. The domain of creating belongs uniquely to God. To manipulate that domain according to human plans is to deny one's fundamental relationship with God as a creature before the Creator. Use of contraception, therefore, does not promote conjugal love but undermines that love because in acting irreverently toward God, one loses sight of the sacred value of marriage, the conjugal act, and the beloved.

Von Hildebrand's repeated claim that use of artificial birth control involves a grave sin of irreverence supports Paul VI's claims that contraception leads to infidelity, destroys respect among spouses, and tempts public authorities to exert undue control over the spousal mission of parenting. Von Hildebrand's analysis also supports John Paul II's critique of the "contraceptive mentality." Nonetheless, while von Hildebrand identifies use of artificial birth control as a grave sin he acknowledges that not all who support contraception do so from the same disposition. He argues that on one extreme some individuals with resentment toward the Church are looking for a chance to undermine the Church's moral authority. However, at the other extreme are those spouses who had been taught that use of artificial birth control is an acceptable means to preventing pregnancy.

For the latter group, von Hildebrand seeks to bring greater clarity to the Church's position on contraception and to clarify the role of conscience in the moral life. He proposes that conscience's role in moral decisions is not to inform about moral behavior but to warn against immoral behavior. Therefore, the central issue concerning artificial birth control is not whether or not one's conscience warns against use of contraception but rather is use of artificial birth control moral and is Paul VI a legitimate authority to speak on the issue?

Von Hildebrand maintains that Pope Paul VI has a teaching authority on matters of faith and morals. This authority was formally exercised in Paul VI's condemnation of artificial birth control in *Humanae vitae*, an encyclical that was long awaited, dramatically pronounced, and in accordance with the unbroken tradition of the Church. Von Hildebrand argues that denial of Paul VI's condemnation is a claim against the Church's teaching authority. Further, in procreation, the Creator uniquely honors spouses by allowing them to participate in His creative power. When spouses use artificial birth control they commit a grave sin of irreverence in that they seek to appropriate power that should be reserved for the Creator.

Notes

1. Pius XI speaks of the need to repeat Church teaching on the issue of artificial birth control, since "openly departing from the uninterrupted Christian tradition some recently have judged it possible solemnly to declare another doctrine regarding this question" (*Casti connubii*, section 56, 28). See also Janet Smith, *Humanae Vitae: A Generation Later* (Washington, D.C.: The Catholic University of America), 5.

2. He writes, "All the more distressing is it for Catholics that, despite the noble general idea, despite the rather Catholic and anti-puritan appreciation of spousal love as belongs to the deepest meaning of marriage, the message fails in such a central point as on the regulation of birth" ("Lambeth-Botschaft, 20, my translation; the German reads as follows: "Umso schmerzlicher ist es für den Katholiken, daß trotz der edlen Gesamtauffassung, trotz der so katholischen

und antipuritanischen Würdigung der ehelichen Liebe als zum tiefsten Sinn der Ehe gehörig, die Botschaft in einem so zentralen Punkt, wie dem der Geburtenregelung versagt").

3. *Humanae vitae*, section 7, paragraph 2, 277.

4. *Purity*, 10.

5. *The Encyclical "Humanae Vitae,"* xi.

6. *The Encyclical "Humanae Vitae,"* 12-13.

7. *Purity*, 10; von Hildebrand makes this claim forty years before Paul VI writes in *Humanae vitae*: "there is an unbreakable connection [*nexu indissolubili*] between the unitive meaning and the procreative meaning [of the conjugal act], and both are inherent in the conjugal act" (*Humanae vitae*, section 12, paragraph 1, 281, brackets in work cited); John Paul II repeats Paul VI's statement in *Familiaris consortio*, section 32, paragraph 3, 60.

8. *The Encyclical "Humanae Vitae,"* 43, italics in work cited.

9. *The Encyclical "Humanae Vitae,"* 43, italics in work cited; see also *Humanae vitae*, section 13, paragraph 1, 281-82.

10. *Man and Woman*, 85; see also *Humanae vitae*, section 16, paragraph 3, 285.

11. "Lambeth-Botschaft," 27; Paul VI makes a similar acknowledgement in *Humanae vitae*: "It cannot be denied that the spouses in each case have, for defensible reasons [*probabiles rationes*], made a mutual and firm decision to avoid having a child; and [it cannot be denied that] each of them is attempting to ensure that a child will not be born" (section 16, paragraph 4, 285; Smith occasionally alters the paragraph distribution as found in *AAS*. This quote is found in paragraph three of *AAS* 60 [1968]: 492).

12. *The Encyclical "Humanae Vitae,"* 41.

13. *The Encyclical "Humanae Vitae,"* 44.

14. *The Encyclical "Humanae Vitae,"* 43; see also 45, where he critiques the position that artificial birth control is merely a biological interference.

15. *The Encyclical "Humanae Vitae,"* 43, italics in work cited.

16. See also *Casti connubii*, sections 55-56, 28-29; Pius XII, 161; and *Humanae vitae*, section 13, paragraphs 2-3 [paragraph 1 in *AAS*], 282; *AAS* 60 (1968): 489.

17. *Marriage*, 23.

18. "Lambeth-Botschaft," 25-26, my translation; the German reads: "eines vermessenen Eingriffs in das Geheimnis der Entstehung eines neuen Menschen . . . die den Charackter eines frevelhaften Eingriffes in gottgewollte Zusammenhänge hat, noch den einer Verletzung des Geheimnisses dieser Sphäre."

19. "Lambeth-Botschaft," 28, my translation; the German reads: "ein frevelhaft freches Verletzen des Geheimnischarakters dieser Sphäre, ein anmaßendes sich als Herr dieses Gebietes Aufspielen, ein unehrfürchtiges Schalten und Walten auf einem Gebiet, das zu den besonderen Reservaten Gottes gehört . . . eine unehrfürchtige Anmaßung Gott gegenüber." See also *Art of Living*, 10.

20. *Man and Woman*, 97-98 and *The Encyclical "Humanae Vitae,"* 35.

21. *The Encyclical "Humanae Vitae,"* 37; see also "Lambeth-Botschaft," 27, *Man and Woman*, 98 and *The Encyclical "Humanae Vitae,"* 36, 47 and 87; von Hildebrand even proposes that the interference of artificial birth control may "throw back into the void a being that God had intended to exist" (*Marriage*, 23). In the latter statement, von Hildebrand seems to go too far since something that does not exist is not a thing at all at least not in the sense that it can be thrown into the void.

22. *The Encyclical "Humanae Vitae,"* 48, footnote 14; to further illustrate the distinction between active intervention and letting things occur von Hildebrand employs the analogy of euthanasia (*The Encyclical "Humanae Vitae,"* 47-48).

23. Von Hildebrand simply notes this position in a footnote to highlight the importance of active intervention versus letting things happen. He does not provide further details about questions of mixed intentions, moral cooperation, or habits of formation. Pius XI seems to maintain a similar position in *Casti connubii*, when he writes that the "Holy Church knows well that not infrequently one of the parties is sinned against rather than sinning, when for a grave cause he or she reluctantly allows the perversion of the right order." Pius XI further explains, however, that "in such a case, there is no sin, provided that, mindful of the law of charity, he or she does not neglect to seek to dissuade and to deter the partner from sin" (section 59, 30).

24. *The Encyclical "Humanae Vitae,"* 72.

25. *The Encyclical "Humanae Vitae,"* 72; Paul VI explains that while "it is sometimes permissible to tolerate moral evil—when it is the lesser evil and when one does so in order that one might avoid a greater evil, or so that one might promote a greater good. It is never permissible, however, to do evil so that good might result, not even for the most serious reasons. . . . Thus, it is a serious error to think that a conjugal act, deprived deliberately [*ex industria*] of its fertility, and which consequently is intrinsically wrong [*intrinsece inhonestum*], can be justified by being grouped together with the fertile acts of the whole of the marriage" (*Humanae vitae*, section 14, paragraph 4, 283-84, brackets in work cited); Paul VI further qualifies this remark by explaining that the Church allows "the use of medical treatment necessary for curing diseases of the body although this treatment may thwart one's ability to procreate. Such treatment is permissible even if the reduction of fertility is foreseen, as long as the infertility is not directly intended for any reason whatsoever" (*Humanae vitae*, section 15, 284).

26. "Lambeth-Botschaft," 28; the German reads as follows: "Diese Haltung ist aber, außer ihrer Sündigkeit an sich, auch unverträglich mit einer Grundvoraussetzung der Reinheit—eben dieser Scheu vor dem Geheimnis, diesem Bewußtsein, nur mit der ausdrücklichen Sanktion Gottes diese Sphäre aktualisieren zu dürfen, diesem ehrfürchtigen Lauschen und Horchen auf Gottes Absichten." See also *Man and Woman*, 98 and *The Encyclical "Humanae Vitae,"* 36). John Paul II makes a similar claim just over fifty years after von Hildebrand's "Lambeth-Botschaft." John Paul II writes that use of contraception harms conjugal love because it prevents a complete gift of self: "When couples, by means of recourse to contraception, separate these two meanings that God the Creator has inscribed in the being of man and woman and in the dynamism of their sexual communion, they act as 'arbiters' of the divine plan and they 'manipulate' and degrade human sexuality—and with it themselves and their married partner—by altering its value of 'total' self-giving. Thus the innate language that expresses the total reciprocal self-giving of husband and wife is overlaid, through contraception, by an objectively contradictory language, namely, that of not giving oneself totally to the other. This leads not only to a positive refusal to be open to life but also to a falsification of the inner truth of conjugal love, which is called upon to give itself in personal totality" (section 32, paragraph 4, 61).

27. *Humanae vitae*, section 17, paragraph 1, 286.

28. *Humanae vitae*, section 17, paragraph 1, 286.

29. *Humanae vitae*, section 17, paragraph 1, 286.

30. *Humanae vitae*, section 17, paragraph 2, 286, brackets in work cited.

31. *Humanae vitae*, section 2, paragraph 1, 273.

32. *Familiaris consortio*, section 6, paragraph 2, 12.

33. *Familiaris consortio*, section 30, paragraph 6, 57.

34. *Familiaris consortio*, section 6, paragraph 4, 13.

35. *Familiaris consortio*, section 30, paragraph 2, 56.

36. *The Encyclical "Humanae Vitae,"* xii-xiii.

37. *The Encyclical "Humanae Vitae,"* xiii.

38. *The Encyclical "Humanae Vitae,"* xiv.

39. *The Encyclical "Humanae Vitae,"* 65; see also von Hildebrand's discussion of value responses in *Ethics*, 191-243.

40. *The Encyclical "Humanae Vitae,"* 65, italics in work cited. Von Hildebrand offers a more focused definition of conscience than the Council Fathers offer in *Gaudium et spes*: "Deep within his conscience man discovers a law which he has not laid upon himself but which he must obey. Its voice, ever calling him to love and to do what is good and to avoid evil, tells him inwardly at the right moment: do this, shun that. For man has in his heart a law inscribed by God. His dignity lies in observing this law, and by it he will be judged. His conscience is man's most secret core, and his sanctuary. There he is alone who voice echoes in his depths" (*Gaudium et spes*, section 16, 916).

41. *The Encyclical "Humanae Vitae,"* 66, italics in work cited.

42. *The Encyclical "Humanae Vitae,"* 68.

43. *The Encyclical "Humanae Vitae,"* 69.

44. *The Encyclical "Humanae Vitae,"* 66.

45. *The Encyclical "Humanae Vitae,"* 66 and 74; see also 82; for more on the necessity of authority, see Yves Simon, *A General Theory of Authority* (Notre Dame: University of Notre Dame Press, 1962).

46. *The Encyclical "Humanae Vitae,"* 75-76; see also 68 and 80. The Fathers of the Second Vatican Council make a similar affirmation about the role of the Church forming the conscience of Catholics: "in forming their consciences the faithful must pay careful attention to the sacred and certain teaching of the Church. For the Catholic Church is by the will of Christ the teacher of truth. It is her duty to proclaim and teach with authority the truth which is Christ and, at the same time, to declare and and confirm by her authority the principles of the moral order which spring from human nature itself" (Vatican II, *Declaration on Religious Freedom*, trans. Lawrence Ryan, in *Vatican Council II: The Conciliar and Post Conciliar Documents*, new rev. ed., ed. Austin Flannery [Collegeville, MN: Liturgical Press, 1975], section 14, paragraph 3, 811). Von Hildebrand explains that the Church's authority "does not extend to such questions as what profession a person should choose, whom he should marry or not marry, except in those cases where canonical obstacles stand in the way" (*The Encyclical "Humanae Vitae,"* 76). While he notes that the Church's authority flows from the guidance of the Holy Spirit, he does not explain further what he means by the Church's "absolute" authority.

47. *The Encyclical "Humanae Vitae,"* 80.

48. *The Encyclical "Humanae Vitae,"* 69.

49. *The Encyclical "Humanae Vitae,"* 69. For further discussion on the topic of conscience, Church teaching, and *Humanae vitae*, see William E. May, "Conscience Formation and the Teaching of the Church," *Homiletic and Pastoral Review* 87, 1 (October 1986): 11-20. This article is re-printed in *Why Humanae Vitae Was Right: A Reader*, ed. Janet E. Smith (San Francisco, CA: Ignatius Press, 1993), 365-82.

50. *The Encyclical "Humanae Vitae,"* 70-71; see also *The Encyclical "Humanae Vitae,"* xiii and von Hildebrand's application of this conclusion in reference to overpopulation in *Man and Woman*, 99-100 and 102. Pius XI similarly condemns use of artificial birth control to prevent pregnancy as an intrinsically evil act: "But no reason, however grave, may be put forward by which anything intrinsically against nature may become conformable to nature and morally good. Since, therefore, the conjugal act is destined primarily by nature for the begetting of children, those who in exercising it deliberately frustrate its natural power and purpose sin against nature and commit a deed which is shameful and intrinsically vicious" (*Casti connubii*, section 54, 28). See Pius XII, who quotes Pius XI's formulation (Pius XII, 167), and Paul VI, who references Pius XI and Pius XII, and makes the same claim (*Humanae vitae*, section 14, paragraph 3, 283; section 14, paragraph 4, 284); John Paul II repeats and summarizes Paul VI's statements in *Familiaris consortio*, section 32, paragraph 3, 60.

51. "Lambeth-Botschaft," 28, my translation; the German reads: "Daher liegt in dem Gebrauch empfängnisverhütender Mittel eine schwere Sünde, die keine noch so berechtigen Motive, wie Gesundheitsrücksichten, oder die wirtschaftliche Unmöglichkeit, Kinder, aufzuziehen, zu etwas Erlaubtem machen können."

Conclusion

Dietrich von Hildebrand is widely acknowledged for contributing to the Catholic tradition's increased recognition of conjugal love's role in marriage. Nonetheless, his published thought on conjugal love, marriage and procreation have received little commentary. While much can be done to introduce his thought to scholarly discussion, one of the first steps in this effort is to present his thought in a systematic fashion. This is particularly necessary for von Hildebrand's works because he uses unique language, language that he does not always clearly define. Further, his way of presenting material is such that he gradually unfolds a topic and returns to it from different angles as he discusses other related themes. Therefore, in order to see his thought systematically, one must pull together the insights he provides throughout his published works.

A. CONJUGAL LOVE, MARRIAGE, AND THE CONJUGAL ACT

A systematic look at von Hildebrand's thought is a rewarding study. His remarks hold together with remarkable consistency and present a powerful whole. For von Hildebrand, the foundation of the moral life is right relationship with God. God has established a created order. Man, in his respect for God, seeks genuine contact with the created world. The world is filled with values, that is, things good in themselves. One must understand the intrinsic values of the world and provide an appropriate response to those values. Such a response is not a programmatic action that can be anticipated and charted. Rather, one must respond with one's intellect, will, and affections as life unfolds. In focusing on the values of God's creation, one cultivates dispositions of reverence before God, gratitude for the values of the world, appreciation for those values, and humility in giving way to things that have intrinsic importance.

Von Hildebrand provides a compelling presentation both of conjugal love as a unique type of love and the sanctification of that love in the Christian context. This love is rooted in genuine contact with the dignity of the beloved. The lover makes the beloved uniquely thematic in his life, that is, the beloved takes priority in the lover's thoughts and in action in a way that one cannot describe simply in terms of the value of things. In conjugal love, this attentiveness to the other is not a one-way street but mutual.

One of the distinguishing features of conjugal love is its unitive character. All types of love involve an intention for union and a benevolent care for the beloved. Unlike parental love, sibling love, love of parents, love of friends, all of which are more directed toward benevolence, conjugal love, like love of God, is directed more toward unity. One who loves conjugally seeks not only the well-being of the beloved but also to unite with the beloved.

This unique unitive love can occur only between a man and a woman. The difference between man and woman is not merely biological but spiritual and metaphysical. Man and woman are two different types of humanity. In their differences, man and woman complement one another and thereby are capable of a unique union. This union entails that the spouses give themselves to one another without reserve.

While conjugal love is the truly authentic motive for marriage and those who have conjugal love will desire marriage, the presence of conjugal love does not make a marriage and the validity of marriage does not require the presence of conjugal love. Marriage is essentially a formal, solemn, and free act in which the spouses commit to fidelity, the fostering of conjugal love, and openness to children. The marriage commitment establishes an objective bond between the spouses that cannot be changed arbitrarily by a new act of the will.

Conjugal love and marriage are transformed in the light of Christ. Conjugal love is rooted in the lover's recognition of the beloved's dignity. In Christ, that dignity is seen with greater clarity. The beloved has unique value as one created by God, one redeemed by Christ, a temple of the Holy Spirit, and destined for eternal fellowship with the Triune God. In Christ, the lover is concerned not only with the general well-being of the beloved but with the beloved's eternal salvation.

Marriage is transformed in Christ in that the motive for marriage becomes not only the actualization of conjugal love but also the conviction that God has destined the beloved to be one's life-long partner on the path to salvation. Marriage involves a commitment to one's spouse but also a commitment to Christ. The cultivation of conjugal love in marriage is a divine service.

Entrance into marriage involves a kind of risk. Since spouses make a lifelong commitment before God, marriage has implications for the eternal salvation of their souls. Von Hildebrand, maintaining the common western view, affirms that the spouses themselves confer the sacrament of marriage. Therefore, spouses should be aware of the commitment they are expressing and should enter marriage only after thoughtful discernment and reflection. God's love should remain central for spouses. In their unique love for one another, they participate in the Love of God and the Love that Christ has for the Church. As a sign of God's enduring and faithful Love, sacramental marriage is indissoluble.

Von Hildebrand's account of conjugal love and marriage sheds light on the conjugal act. He explains that the conjugal act is intended by God for the actualization of conjugal love and the consummation of marriage. As the consummation of marriage, the conjugal act renders sacramental marriage indissoluble. Just as spouses should enter marriage only in accordance with God's will so also spouses should express the conjugal act only with God's sanction. As the actualization of conjugal love, the conjugal act should express concern for the beloved's well-being, intention for union, the giving of one's self without reserve, and an exclusive belonging to the beloved.

The conjugal act, therefore, is a spiritual act that is essentially deep. The spouses either express the action with God's sanction, in the context of marriage, and with the intention of actualizing their conjugal love or they disregard God's intentions and violate the gift and mystery of marriage and conjugal love. Von Hildebrand warns against the misuse of the conjugal act. He explains that sexual desire and the human body's dynamic orientation toward sexual union reflect the depth of the action. As a result, spouses must be prepared to express the action as a deep actualization of conjugal love or they risk losing themselves to their own vital-corporeality.

B. THE PRIMARY MEANING AND END OF MARRIAGE

In his early work on *Marriage*, von Hildebrand proposed that conjugal love is the primary meaning of marriage even while procreation is the primary end. A number of those who review the English translation of this work critique von Hildebrand's lack of clarity in distinguishing between his central terms, "meaning" and "end." While von Hildebrand does not explicitly define "meaning" and "end," a systematic analysis of the topic reveals how he implicitly distinguishes the terms.

Since von Hildebrand receives criticism for his use of the term "primary meaning," one does well to recognize what von Hildebrand does not mean by the phrase. Meaning is not merely a subjective, passive feeling. Conjugal love is not primary in the sense that conjugal love is whatever one makes it out to be and therefore marriage is whatever one makes it out to be. Rather, conjugal love is the primary, created meaning of marriage. One can understand the primacy of conjugal love only in relation to God.

Conjugal love is not the ontological essence of marriage. While one must foster conjugal love after entering marriage, the presence of conjugal love is not required for marriage to be valid. Conjugal love also is not primary to marriage as an end. Rather, conjugal love is primary as the truly authentic motivation for marriage and as the ongoing vitality of marriage.

One can understand von Hildebrand's remarks on procreation only in light of the principle of superabundance and the virtue of reverence. He distinguishes the principle of superabundance from instrumental finality. He explains that in some cases the means-end relationship is such that the significance of the means is completely dependent on and reduced to the end. This is instrumental finality. In other cases, the means has a unique value on its own regardless of whether it leads to an end and even when it leads to an end. In this case, the thing that *can* serve as a means to an end is not reduced to its role as a means. The means has value and the end flows superabundantly from that value. This is superabundant finality. Von Hildebrand describes the end of procreation as a superabundant fruit of the conjugal act, which has unique meaning as an actualization of conjugal love. Procreation does not result from every expression of the conjugal act and when it does, it results not instrumentally but superabundantly.

Von Hildebrand argues that reverence is a foundational virtue not only for procreation but for the moral life in general. Reverence relates to one's fundamental disposition before God and therefore one's basic stance before God's creation. Reverence has particular bearing on the topic of procreation which involves the creation of human life. Only God is Creator; only He can create out of nothing. While God honors spouses by allowing them to participate in His creative power, the domain of creating belongs uniquely to the Creator. Procreation, in a unique way, brings spouses face to face with God. They are reminded that He alone is Creator but also that He desires to share His Divine life with humanity. Procreation is the primary end of marriage because it is a superabundant end that deals with man's fundamental relationship with God as a creature before the Loving Creator.

Von Hildebrand's emphasis on conjugal love does not diminish procreation's role in marriage but enhances and clarifies that role. His account of conjugal love clarifies procreation's role because he demonstrates that marriage and the conjugal act have significance in addition to procreation. Spouses should not enter marriage in order to use their spouse to attain children. Further, while spouses who are capable of having children must be open to procreation, the validity of a marriage does not require that spouses actually receive the blessing of children.

Von Hildebrand explains the fruit of procreation from the top down. That is, he begins with God's love and then identifies conjugal love and marriage as a participation and manifestation of that love. Conjugal love committed in marriage bears spiritual fruit by promoting personal conversion and thereby leading each spouse to eternal paradise. From this spiritually fruitful relationship flows the superabundant fruit of procreation. Von Hildebrand's focus is not to describe the fruitfulness of conjugal love or the superabundance of God's love in terms of procreation but rather to explain the fruit of procreation in terms of both God's love and conjugal love committed in marriage.

Von Hildebrand's account of conjugal love enhances procreation's role in marriage. He describes conjugal love, marriage, and the conjugal act in terms of reverence for God and His created order. If spouses reverently discern conjugal love, their vocation to marriage and God's sanction in expressing the conjugal act, then they will be disposed to stand reverently before the Creator concerning procreation. Further, the fact that procreation is a superabundant fruit of conjugal love testifies that God's Love stands at the foundation of all creation. Procreation is not merely a biological consequence of sexual intercourse but the fruit of a profound love shared between spouses and the more profound Love of God, who alone creates every human soul.

C. THE RHYTHM METHOD AND ARTIFICIAL BIRTH CONTROL

In his article "Lambeth-Conference" and his short book, *The Encyclical "Humanae Vitae,"* von Hildebrand applies his analysis of procreation to the rhythm method and artificial birth control. Although he says little about the good of children and the parenting mission of marriage, von Hildebrand provides a rich framework for such reflection.

The relationship between the conjugal act and procreation is a profoundly deep and mysterious connection that should not be altered because it is divinely established by the Creator, the value of all values. God alone is Creator and He has uniquely honored spouses by allowing them to participate in His creative power. Those spouses who have serious reasons for postponing pregnancy may avoid pregnancy through recourse to the rhythm method. That is, through attentiveness to the divinely established connection between the conjugal act and procreation, they may express the conjugal act when procreation is not likely to result. The rhythm method is an acceptable means to postpone pregnancy for two reasons. First, since the conjugal act is a spiritual act spouses must decide when and when not to express the action. Second, spouses leave intact the manner in which the Creator has connected the conjugal act with procreation.

The abstinence required by the rhythm method does not place an undue burden on spouses. All Christians are called to make sacrifices and spouses often abstain from expressing the conjugal act during business trips. They should, therefore, have no problem doing so for the sake of their spouse and their family. The rhythm method does not harm conjugal love because abstinence can encourage other expressions of love and can purify the spouses' intentions for expressing the conjugal act.

Spousal use of artificial birth control to prevent pregnancy, however, is a grave sin of irreverence. Spouses, by manipulating how God allows them to participate in His work of creation, subvert the relationship between creature and Creator and appropriate power that should be reserved to God alone. Since reverence is the foundation of the moral life, use of artificial birth control does not promote but undermines authentic expression of conjugal love. Conjugal love and procreation, therefore, should not be pitted against one another; rather, both are essential to the conjugal act.

Von Hildebrand critiques those who affirm that artificial birth control should be determined by the conscience of the spouses. The primary question, he argues, is whether or not artificial birth control is immoral. Further, since one's conscience is formed in relation to statements of legitimate authorities, Catholics should adhere to Paul VI's condemnation of artificial birth control as found in the encyclical, *Humanae vitae*.

D. TOPICS FOR FURTHER STUDY

I have not attempted to deal exhaustively with topics indirectly related to von Hildebrand's analysis of procreation and certainly not as relates to his remarks on conjugal love, marriage, and the conjugal act. Although his published writings on conjugal love already have received some public recognition, his works and the topics discussed in them remain a rich ground deserving of more consideration.

While von Hildebrand is recognized for contributing to the Catholic tradition's growing appreciation of conjugal love, more work could be done to identify remarks on conjugal love that preceded von Hildebrand's analysis. The "primary meaning" of marriage certainly had numerous anticipations in the tradition. What enabled von Hildebrand to contribute on the topic of conjugal love is also worth more consideration. In particular, how did his understanding of the affections, the dignity of women and his phenomenological background influence his insights?

His analysis of the conjugal act as a spiritual act merits further study. His discussion on the way in which the conjugal act is ordered to procreation and his emphasis on the conjugal act as an actualization of conjugal love, with its characteristic mutuality, permanence, exclusivity, and unity, offer terminological distinctions that help clarify how the conjugal act is distinct from premarital intercourse, rape, incest, acts of masturbation, and homosexual acts.

The Catholic tradition would benefit from a comparison between von Hildebrand and other influential thinkers. A project certain to bear great fruit would be a comparison between von Hildebrand's writings with those of Karol Wojtyla/John Paul II. They both have a phenomenological background, they are attentive to the personalist values of marriage, they share an appreciation for beauty and art, and they have written a good deal about marriage and sexual ethics. One could evaluate how their writings compare with one another but also if and how von Hildebrand influences John Paul II's work, especially since John Paul II, like von Hildebrand, is not always good about citing his sources.

I have tried to highlight some parallels between von Hildebrand and Augustine in footnotes. The relationship between these two thinkers on marriage and sexual ethics is fascinating. Von Hildebrand highlights his affinity with Augustine in their mutual emphasis on the affections. And yet, von Hildebrand's attentiveness to the affections is what in part enables him to see the importance of conjugal love and thereby separate himself from Augustine's insistence that procreation is the only legitimate motivation for expressing the conjugal act.

Von Hildebrand offers a rich discussion on the meaning of infertile marriages. He argues that couples who are infertile may have a fulfilling marriage insofar as they actualize their love for one another and draw on the sacramental graces of marriage to assist one another on their path to eternal fellowship with God. Do spouses who know they are infertile have to express in their wedding vows openness to children? If so, what are they expressing?

More study could be done on the mission of parenting and the discernment of family size. Von Hildebrand's work would be furthered by an analysis of what constitutes serious reasons for postponing children. Such analysis is even more necessary now that methods of natural family planning have reached unprecedented levels of precision in the prevention of pregnancy.

Central to von Hildebrand's account of procreation is the principle of superabundance and reverence. A further analysis of superabundance in relation to discussion of procreation found in Augustine, Aquinas, and Church documents would help to locate von Hildebrand in the tradition. Further, how does von Hildebrand's analysis of superabundance relate to Bonaventure's discussion of the same theme? If reverence is central for marriage and procreation, then how might one promote reverence for conjugal love, marriage, the conjugal act, and procreation? How does the liturgy for sacramental marriages actualize or fail to actualize reverence for marriage and procreation? How might von Hildebrand's remarks on reverence apply to contemporary discussion of assisted reproductive technologies (A.R.T.)?

Reverence places humanity before its Creator as creatures before a Loving God. Like the mysteries of creation and the Incarnation, procreation deals with superabundant love and the intersection of the Infinite with the finite.

God creates all things out of nothing, including humanity, whom He creates in His image. God becomes man and dies for man to fully reveal Himself and thereby overcomes the separation that exists between Creator and creature. And in procreation, He honors spouses by allowing them to participate in His creation of new life as an actualization of His Love: "O Lord our God, who created man pure and spotless and thereafter ordained that in the propagation of the human race one generation should be produced from another by the *mystery of sweet love*."[1]

Note

1. *Purity*, 15, italics in work cited; von Hildebrand repeats this wedding prayer in *Marriage*, 22 and *The Encyclical "Humanae Vitae,"* 41. In both *Purity* and *Marriage*, von Hildebrand indicates that he read this quote in a work by Wintersig entitled "Liturgie und Frauenseele," and in *Marriage*, he further indicates that Wintersig is quoting from the *Sacramentum Fuldense*.

Bibliography

Aquinas, Thomas. *Treatise on Happiness*. Translated by John A. Oesterle. Notre Dame, Indiana: University of Notre Dame Press, 1964.

Arjonillo, Rolando B. *Conjugal Love of the Ends of Marriage: A Study of Dietrich von Hildebrand and Herbert Doms in the Light of the Pastoral Constitution 'Gaudium et Spes.'* Bern: Lang, 1998.

Augustine. *City of God*. Translated by Henry Bettenson. London: Penguin Books, 1984.

______. *On the Good of Marriage*. Translated by C. L. Cornish. In *Nicene and Post-Nicene Fathers*. Vol. 3. Edited by Philip Schaff. Peabody, Massachusetts: Hendrickson, 1994.

Bruehl, C. Review of *Marriage*, by Dietrich von Hildebrand. *Commonweal* 36 (26 June 1942): 234.

Code of Canon Law, Latin-English Translation: New English Translation. Translated by Canon Law Society of America. Washington, D.C.: Canon Law Society of America, 1999.

Dimpfl, Maria. "Das Wesen der ehelichen Liebe in Werken Dietrich von Hildebrands." Thes., Pontificia Università Lateranense, 1992/93.

Doms, Herbert. *Vom Sinn und Zweck der Ehe*. Breslau: Ostdeutsche Verlagsanstalt, 1935. Translated by George Sayer as *The Meaning of Marriage*. London: Sheed and Ward, 1939.

Dore, F. J. Review of *In Defense of Purity*, by Dietrich von Hildebrand. *Thought* 7, 2 (September 1932): 325-27.

Elliott, Peter. *What God Has Joined . . . The Sacramentality of Marriage*. Staten Island, New York: Alba House, 1990.

Ford, John C. and Gerard Kelly. *Marriage Questions*. Vol. 2 of *Contemporary Moral Theology*. Westminster, Maryland: Newman Press, 1964.

Ford, John C. Review of *Marriage*, by Dietrich von Hildebrand. *Thought* 17 (September 1942): 544-45.

______. *The Validity of Virginal Marriage*. Worcester, Massachusetts: Harrigan Press, 1938.

Gemmel, J. Review of *Reinheit und Jungfräulichkeit*, by Dietrich von Hildebrand. *Scholastik* 2 (1927): 478-79.

Grabowski, John S. "Person or Nature? Rival Personalisms in 20th Century Catholic Sexual Ethics," *Studia Moralia* 35 (1997): 283-312.

______. *Sex and Virtue: An Introduction to Sexual Ethics*. Washington, D.C.: The Catholic University of America Press, 2003.

Gierens, M. Review of *Die Ehe*, by Dietrich von Hildebrand. *Stimmen der Zeit* 119 (1930): 386.

G.L.D. Review of *Marriage*, by Dietrich von Hildebrand. *Oratre Fratres* 16 (14 June 1941): 382.

Grubb, Geoffrey. "The Anthropology of Marriage in Significant Roman Catholic Documents from *Casti Connubii* to *Gaudium et Spes* (Doms, Hildebrand)." PhD diss., Saint Louis University, 1986.

Hardon, John A. Review of *Man and Woman*, by Dietrich von Hildebrand. *Review for Religious* 25 (1966): 1119.

Hennrich, Kilian. Review of *Marriage*, by Dietrich von Hildebrand. *Homiletic and Pastoral Review* 42 (1942): 1078.

Hewitt, Robert A. Review of *Marriage*, by Dietrich von Hildebrand. *America* 67 (6 June 1942): 244.

Janssen, A. Review of *Die Ehe*, by Dietrich von Hildebrand. *Ephemerides theologicae Lovanienses* 7 (1931): 601.

John Paul II. *Familiaris Consortio*. Translated by Vatican Press. In *The Post-Synodal Apostolic Exhortations of John Paul II*, edited by J. Michael Miller, 148-233. Huntington, Indiana: Our Sunday Visitor, 1998. *AAS* 74 (1982): 81-191.

______. *Man and Woman He Created Them: A Theology of the Body*. Translated by Michael Waldstein. Boston, Massachusetts: Pauline Books, 2006.

Kurz, Edelbert. Review of *Reinheit und Jungfräulichkeit*, by Dietrich von Hildebrand. *Katechetische Blätter* 29 (1928): 451-54.

Lamalle, E. Review of *Die Ehe*, by Dietrich von Hildebrand. *Nouvelle revue théologique* 57 (1930): 527.

Leo XIII. *Arcanum Divinae Sapientiae*. Translator anonymous. In *The Papal Encyclicals: 1878-1903*, edited by Claudia Carlen, IHM, 29-40. Ann Arbor, Michigan: Pierian Press, 1990. *AAS* 12 (1879/80): 385-402.

Lonergan, Bernard. Review of *Marriage*, by Dietrich von Hildebrand. In *Shorter Papers*, 153-56. Vol. 20 of *Collected Works of Bernard Lonergan*. Edited by Frederick Crowe and Robert Doran. Toronto: University of Toronto Press, 2007.

Mackin, Theodore, S.J., *What Is Marriage?* New York: Paulist Press, 1982.

Marra, William A. "Von Hildebrand on Love, Happiness, and Sex." In *The Catholic Writer*, edited by Ralph McInerny, 119-27. San Francisco, California: Ignatius Press, 1991.

Mouton, Michelle. *From Nurturing the Nation to Purifying the Volk: Weimar and Nazi Family Policy, 1918-1945*. New York: Cambridge University Press, 2007.

M.P.B. Review of *Marriage*, by Dietrich von Hildebrand. *Dominicana* 27 (October 1942): 189.

Noonan, John T., Jr. *Contraception: A History of Its Treatment by the Catholic Theologians and Canonists*. 2nd ed. Cambridge, Massachusetts: Harvard University Press, 1986.

Olson, Carl. Review of *Man, Woman, and the Meaning of Love*, by Dietrich von Hildebrand. *National Catholic Register* 78, 34 (August 25-31 2002): 14.

Paul VI. *Humanae Vitae*. Encyclical letter. Translated by Janet Smith. In *Humanae Vitae: A Generation Later*, 272-95. Washington, D.C.: The Catholic University of America Press, 1991. *AAS* 60 (1968): 481-503.

Peters, Edward, trans. *The 1917 Pio-Benedictine Code of Canon Law*. San Francisco, California: Ignatius Press, 2001.

Pius XI. *Casti Connubii*. Encyclical letter. Vatican translation. Boston, Massachusetts: St. Paul Editions. *AAS* 22 (1930): 539-92, 604.

Pius XII. *Selected Addresses*. Vol. 1 of *The Major Addresses of Pope Pius XII*. Edited by Vincent A. Yzermans. St. Paul, Minnesota: North Central, 1961. *AAS* 43 (1951): 835-54.

Ryan, John A. "The Moral Aspects of Periodical Continence." *Ecclesiastical Review* 89 (1933): 28-39.

______. Review of *Man and Woman*, by Dietrich von Hildebrand. *Theological Studies* 27 (1966): 473-75.

Schmiedeler, Edgar. Review of *Marriage*, by Dietrich von Hildebrand. *The Catholic Educational Review* 40 (October 1942): 509.

Schmitt, Albert. Review of *Die Ehe*, by Dietrich von Hildebrand. *Zeitschrift für katholische Theologie* 54 (1930): 309.

Schneider, E. Review of *Die Ehe*, by Dietrich von Hildebrand. *Theologie und Glaube* 21 (1929): 813.

Schwarz, Balduin V., ed. *The Human Person and the World of Values: A Tribute to Dietrich von Hildebrand by His Friends in Philosophy*. New York, New York: Fordham University Press, 1960.

Seifert, Josef. "Dietrich von Hildebrands philosophische Entdeckung der 'Wertantwort' und die Grundlegung der Ethik." *Aletheia* 5 (1992): 34-58.

Shannon, William H. *The Lively Debate: Response to 'Humanae Vitae.'* New York: Sheed and Ward, 1970.

Slade, Francis. "Ends and Purposes." In *Final Causality in Nature and Human Affairs*. Edited by Richard F. Hassing, 83-84. Washington, D.C.: The Catholic University of America Press, 1997.

Smith, Janet. *Humanae Vitae: A Generation Later*. Washington, D.C.: The Catholic University of America Press, 1991.

______, ed. *Why Humanae Vitae Was Right: A Reader*. San Francisco, California: Ignatius Press, 1993.

Sośnicka, Joanna. "What Is the Essence of Love? Philosophical Analysis Based on the Thought of Dietrich von Hildebrand." PhD diss., Internationale Akademie für Philosophie im Fürstentum Liechtenstein, 2005.

Umberg, Joh. B. Review of *Reinheit und Jungfräulichkeit*, by Dietrich von Hildebrand. *Zeitschrift für katholische Theologie* 52 (1928): 470.

Vatican Council II. *Gaudium et Spes*. Translated by Ronan Lennon, O.Carm. and Ambrose McNicholl, O.P. In *Vatican Council II: The Conciliar and Post Conciliar Documents*, rev. ed., edited by Austin Flannery, O.P., 903-1001. Collegeville, Minnesota: Liturgical Press, 1975. *AAS* 58 (1966): 1025-1120.

Von Hildebrand, Alice. "Aristotle: The Philosopher," *Logos* 8, 3 (Summer 2005): 112-22.

______. "The Meaning and Purpose of Marriage," *Homiletic and Pastoral Review* (August/September 2008): 24-31.

______. *The Soul of a Lion: Dietrich von Hildebrand*. San Francisco, California: Ignatius Press, 2000.

Von Hildebrand, Dietrich. *Celibacy and the Crisis of Faith*. Translated by John F. Crosby. Chicago: Franciscan Herald Press, 1971. Originally published as *Zölibat und Glaubenskrise*. Regensburg: Josef Habbel, 1970.

______. *Christian Ethics*. New York: David McKay, 1953.

______. *The Encyclical 'Humanae Vitae': A Sign of Contradiction. An Essay on Birth Control and Catholic Conscience*. Translated by Damian Fedoryka and John Crosby. Chicago: Franciscan Herald Press, 1969. Originally published as *Die Enzyklika "Humanae Vitae": ein Zeichen des Widerspruchs*. Regensburg: Josef Habbel, 1968.

______. "Die Idee der sittlichen Handlung," *Jahrbuch für Philosophie und phänomenologische Förschung*, 3 (1916): 126-251.

______. "Lambeth-Botschaft." *Religiöse Besinnung* 4, 1 (1931/32): 20-29. Re-printed in *Die Menschheit am Scheideweg: Gesammelte Abhandlungen und Vorträge*, ed. Karla Mertens, 146-57. Regensburg: Josef Habbel, 1955.

______. *Liturgy and Personality*. Rev. ed. Translated by an anonymous author. Baltimore, Maryland: Helicon Press, 1960. Originally published as *Liturgie und Persönlichkeit*. Salzburg: Anton Pustet, 1933.

______. *Man and Woman*. Chicago: Franciscan Herald Press, 1966.

______. *Marriage*. Translated by Dietrich von Hildebrand, Emmanuel Chapman, and Daniel Sullivan. London: Longmans, Green, 1942. Originally published as *Die Ehe*. Munich: Verlag Ars Sacra, 1929.

______. *Memoiren und Aufsätze gegen den Nationalsozialismus*. Edited by Ernst Wenisch, Rudolf Ebneth and Alice von Hildebrand. Mainz: Matthias-Grünewald, 1994.

______. *Die Menschheit am Scheideweg: Gesammelte Abhandlungen und Vorträge*. Edited by Karla Mertens. Regensburg: Josef Habbel, 1955.

______. *Metaphysik der Gemeinschaft: Untersuchungen über Wesen und Wert der Gemeinschaft*. Vol. 4 of *Dietrich von Hildebrand Gesammelte Werke*. Edited by Dietrich von Hildebrand Gesellschaft. Regensburg: Josef Habbel, 1975. Originally published as *Metaphysik der Gemeinschaft: Untersuchungen über Wesen und Wert der Gemeinschaft*. Augsburg: Haas & Grabherr, 1930.

______. *The Nature of Love*. Translated by John F. Crosby. South Bend, Indiana: St. Augustine's Press, 2009. Originally published as *Das Wesen der Liebe*. Vol. 3 of *Dietrich von Hildebrand Gesammelte Werke*. Edited by Dietrich von Hildebrand Gesellschaft. Regensburg: Josef Habbel, 1971.

______. *Purity: The Mystery of Christian Sexuality*. Translated by an anonymous author. Steubenville, Ohio: Franciscan University Press, 1989. Originally published as *Reinheit und Jungfräulichkeit*. Cologne: Oratoriums Verlag, 1927.

______. *Transformation in Christ: On the Christian Attitude*. Translated by an anonymous author. San Francisco, California: Ignatius Press, 2001. Originally published as Peter Ott [Dietrich von Hildebrand]. *Die Umgestaltung in Christus: Über christliche Grundhaltung*. Einsiedeln: Benziger, 1944.

Von Hildebrand, Dietrich and Alice von Hildebrand. *The Art of Living*. 2nd ed. Manchester, New Hampshire: Sophia Institute Press, 1965.

Von Hildebrand, Dietrich and William A. Marra. *Sex Education: The Basic Issues*. St. Paul, Minnesota: Wanderer Press, 1969.

Waldstein, Michael, "Dietrich von Hildebrand and St. Thomas Aquinas on Goodness and Happiness," *Nova et Vetera* 1, 2 (2003): 403-64.

Wojtyla, Karol. *Love and Responsibility*. Translated by H. T. Willetts. San Francisco, California: Ignatius Press, 1993.

Adolf Pries provided an extensive list of von Hildebrand's works and secondary literature related to those works in the journal Aletheia *5 (1992): 363-430. Preis presents von Hildebrand's works in chronological order and includes translations of those works. The Dietrich von Hildebrand Legacy Project continues to update this bibliography on its website, www.hildebrandlegacy.org.*

Index

About the Author

Kevin Schemenauer is an assistant professor of theology at Marian University in Indianapolis, Indiana. He received an M.A. in historical/systematic theology and a Ph.D. in moral theology/ethics both from The Catholic University of America. His research focuses on marriage and sexual ethics, fundamental moral theology, and Catholic social teaching.

www.ingramcontent.com/pod-product-compliance
Ingram Content Group UK Ltd.
Pitfield, Milton Keynes, MK11 3LW, UK
UKHW041122071026
15587UKWH00009B/92

9 780739 147061